ICOG – Campus
OVARY
Recent Developments and Current Practice

ICOG – Campus
OVARY
Recent Developments and Current Practice

Editors

Uday Thanawala
MBBS MD DGO FCPS DNB
Thanawala Maternity Home and IVF Centre
Navi Mumbai, Maharashtra, India
Chairman, ICOG
Treasurer PCOS Society (India)
Vice President, FOGSI (2015)
Chairperson, Medical Disorders
Committee of FOGSI (2006–2008)
Founder Secretary & Past President, NMOGS

Ashok Kumar
MD PHD
Director Professor and Head
Department of Obstetrics and Gynecology
Atal Bihari Vajpayee Institute of Medical
Sciences and Dr Ram Manohar
Lohia Hospital
New Delhi, India
Honorary Secretary, ICOG (2021–23)

Guest Editor

Madhuri Patil
MD DGO FCPS DFP FICOG
Clinical Director
Dr Patil's Fertility and Endoscopy Clinic
Bengaluru, Karnataka, India
President and Founder Member
Fertility Preservation Society of India (FPSI)
Vice President, Indian Society for Assisted Reproduction (ISAR)
Vice-President and Founder Member, PCOS Society (India)
Associate Editor, Fertility and Sterility
Chairperson, ASPIRE SIG Reproductive Endocrinology
Board Member, Asian Society for Fertility Preservation (ASFP)
Editorial Board Member, Endocrine Society 2020 and 2021
Associate Editor, The Onco Fertility Journal, Official Journal of FPSI
Governing Council Member, ICOG (2021–2023)
Editor-in-Chief, Journal of Human Reproductive Sciences (2013–2020)
Founder President, Karnataka Chapter of Indian Society for Assisted Reproduction

Forewords

S Shantha Kumari, Uday Thanawala

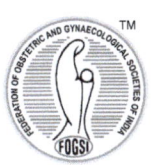 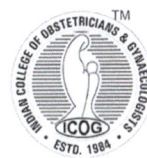

**Indian College of
Obstetricians & Gynaecologists**

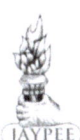

JAYPEE BROTHERS MEDICAL PUBLISHERS
The Health Sciences Publisher
New Delhi | London

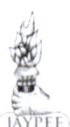 **Jaypee Brothers Medical Publishers (P) Ltd**

Headquarters
Jaypee Brothers Medical Publishers (P) Ltd
EMCA House, 23/23-B
Ansari Road, Daryaganj
New Delhi 110 002, India
Landline: +91-11-23272143, +91-11-23272703
+91-11-23282021, +91-11-23245672
Email: jaypee@jaypeebrothers.com

Corporate Office
Jaypee Brothers Medical Publishers (P) Ltd
4838/24, Ansari Road, Daryaganj
New Delhi 110 002, India
Phone: +91-11-43574357
Fax: +91-11-43574314
Email: jaypee@jaypeebrothers.com

Overseas Office
JP Medical Ltd
83 Victoria Street, London
SW1H 0HW (UK)
Phone: +44 20 3170 8910
Fax: +44 (0)20 3008 6180
Email: info@jpmedpub.com

Website: www.jaypeebrothers.com
Website: www.jaypeedigital.com

© 2023, Jaypee Brothers Medical Publishers

The views and opinions expressed in this book are solely those of the original contributor(s)/author(s) and do not necessarily represent those of editor(s) or publisher of the book.

All rights reserved. No part of this publication may be reproduced, stored or transmitted in any form or by any means, electronic, mechanical, photocopying, recording or otherwise, without the prior permission in writing of the publishers.

All brand names and product names used in this book are trade names, service marks, trademarks or registered trademarks of their respective owners. The publisher is not associated with any product or vendor mentioned in this book.

Medical knowledge and practice change constantly. This book is designed to provide accurate, authoritative information about the subject matter in question. However, readers are advised to check the most current information available on procedures included and check information from the manufacturer of each product to be administered, to verify the recommended dose, formula, method and duration of administration, adverse effects and contraindications. It is the responsibility of the practitioner to take all appropriate safety precautions. Neither the publisher nor the author(s)/editor(s) assume any liability for any injury and/or damage to persons or property arising from or related to use of material in this book.

This book is sold on the understanding that the publisher is not engaged in providing professional medical services. If such advice or services are required, the services of a competent medical professional should be sought.

Every effort has been made where necessary to contact holders of copyright to obtain permission to reproduce copyright material. If any have been inadvertently overlooked, the publisher will be pleased to make the necessary arrangements at the first opportunity.

Inquiries for bulk sales may be solicited at: jaypee@jaypeebrothers.com

ICOG – Campus Ovary: Recent Developments and Current Practice

First Edition: **2023**

ISBN: 978-93-5696-089-3

Printed at:

FOGSI-ICOG OFFICE BEARERS

Dr S Shantha Kumari
President, FOGSI

Dr Madhuri Patel
Secretary General, FOGSI

Dr Uday Thanawala
Chairperson, ICOG

Dr Laxmi Shrikhande
Chairperson Elect

Dr Parag Biniwale
Vice Chairperson, ICOG

Dr Parul Kotdawala
Vice Chairperson Designate

Professor Ashok Kumar
Secretary, ICOG

PAST CHAIRPERSONS

Late Dr CL Jhaveri 1989–96	Late Dr Behram Anklesaria 2011	Dr Mala Arora 2017
Late Dr CS Dawn 1997–99	Dr AK Debdas 2012	Dr S Shantha Kumari 2018
Dr Mahendra N Parikh 2000–02	Dr Hiralal Konar 2013	Professor Tushar Kar 2019
Dr Rohit V Bhatt 2003–05	Dr Atul Munshi 2014	Dr Mandakini Megh 2020–21
Dr Usha B Saraiya 2006–08	Dr Dilip Kumar Dutta 2015	
Dr Duru Shah 2009–10	Professor Krishnendu Gupta 2016	

PAST SECRETARIES FOR THE PERIOD OF 10 YEARS

Dr Sanjay Gupte 2006–08	Dr Jaideep Malhotra 2012–14	Dr Parag Biniwale 2018–21
Dr Hema Divakar 2009–11	Dr S Shantha Kumari 2015–17	

ICOG GOVERNING COUNCIL MEMBERS 2021–2023

Dr Abha Rani Sinha	Dr Fessy Louis	Dr Ranjana Khanna
Dr Alka Pandey	Dr Hafizur Rahman	Dr Reena Wani
Dr Archana Baser	Dr Haresh Doshi	Dr Sarita Bhalerao
Dr Ashis Kumar Mukhopadhyay	Dr Kiran Pandey	Dr Sheela Mane
Dr Ashwini Bhalerao Gandhi	Dr Madhuri Patil	Dr Shobha N Gudi
Dr Aswath Kumar	Dr Mala Srivastava	Dr Sneha Bhuyar
Dr Bhagyalaxmi Nayak	Dr N Palaniappan	Dr Vidya Thobbi
Dr Bharti Maheshwari	Dr Neerja Bhatla	
Dr Charmila Ayyavoo	Dr Pratik Tambe	

Contributors

Anshu Baser
MBBS MS (Gold Medalist) DNB
Consultant
Obstetrician and Gynecology
Akash Hospital
Indore, Madhya Pradesh, India

Archana Baser MS DNB FRCOG FICOG
Director and Unit Head
Department of Obstetrics, Gynecology
and IVF
Akash Hospital
Indore, Madhya Pradesh, India

Ashwini Bhalerao Gandhi
MD DGO DFP FCPS DNB FICOG
Consultant Gynecologist
PD Hinduja Hospital and Hinduja
Healthcare Surgical
Mumbai, Maharashtra, India

Chaitanya Shembekar
MD FICOG FICMCH
Director
Omega Hospitals
Nagpur, Maharashtra, India

Duru Shah MD FRCOG FCPS FICS FICOG
DGO DFP FICMCH
Director
Gynaecworld—the Center for Women's
Health and Fertility
Mumbai, Maharashtra, India

Fessy Louis T MBBS DGO DNB
(Obs & Gyne) FICOG MICOG
Senior Consultant and Associate
Professor
Department of Reproductive Medicine
and Surgery
Amrita Fertility Centre
Amrita Institute of Medical Sciences
Kochi, Kerala, India

Jiteeka Thakkar
MBBS DGO
Infertility Specialist
Laparoscopic Surgeon (Obs and Gyne)
Obstetrician Consultant
Bloom IVF
Mumbai, Maharashtra, India

Jwal Banker
MS (Obs and Gyne)
NOVA IVF Fertility
Ahmedabad, Gujarat, India

Madhuri Patil
MD DGO FCPS DFP FICOG
Clinical Director
Dr Patil's Fertility and Endoscopy Clinic
Bengaluru, Karnataka, India
President and Founder Member
Fertility Preservation Society of India
(FPSI)
Vice President, Indian Society for
Assisted Reproduction (ISAR)
Vice-President and Founder Member
PCOS Society (India)
Associate Editor, Fertility and Sterility
Chairperson, ASPIRE SIG Reproductive
Endocrinology
Board Member, Asian Society for
Fertility Preservation (ASFP)
Editorial Board Member, Endocrine
Society 2020 and 2021
Associate Editor, The Onco Fertility
Journal, Official Journal of FPSI
Governing Council Member
ICOG (2021–2023)
Editor-in-Chief, Journal of Human
Reproductive Sciences (2013–2020)
Founder President, Karnataka
Chapter of Indian Society for Assisted
Reproduction

Contributors

Meenu Handa MS (Obs & Gyne)
DNB (Obs & Gyne) FICOG
Infertility Specialist
Department of Obstetrics
and Gynecology
Fortis Bloom IVF Centre
Fortis Memorial Research Institute
Gurugram, Haryana, India

Meera Ravi Kumar MD
Consultant
Department of Obstetrics
and Gynecology
Amala Institute of Medical Sciences
and Research
Kochi, Kerala, India

Nandita Palshetkar MD FCPS FICOG
FRCOG (UK)
Infertility Specialist
Palshetkar Patil Nursing Home
Mumbai, Maharashtra, India
Lilavati Hospital's Bloom IVF
Centre, Bandra
DY Patil Hospital's Bloom IVF
Centre, Navi Mumbai
La Femme Fortis Bloom IVF
New Delhi, India
Fortis Bloom IVF Centre at Fortis
Hospital, Chandigarh
Bloom IVF Centre, Nashik

Padma Rekha Jirge MRCOG (UK)
FICOG MBA (Health Care Management) PG
DMLE (Med Law & Ethics)
IVF Specialist
Scientific Director
Shreyas Hospital and Sushrut-assisted
Conception Clinic
Kolhapur, Maharashtra, India

Parul Kotdawala MBBS MD (Obs & Gyne)
Endoscopy Surgeon
Department of Obstetrics
and Gynecology
VS Hospital and NHL Municipal
Medical College
Ahmedabad, Gujarat, India

Pratik Tambe MBBS DGO FICOG
ART Consultant and Gynecological
Endoscopic Surgeon
Ashirwad IVF
Mumbai, Maharashtra, India

Priya Vora MBBS MD (Obs & Gyne)
DGO DFP
Consultant
Dr Vora's Maternity Hospital
Mumbai, Maharashtra, India

Rajeshwari Khyade MBBS DGO DNB
Associate Professor
Department of Obstetrics
and Gynecology
Srinivas Institute of Medical Sciences
and Research Centre
Mangaluru, Karnataka, India
Consultant
Gynecologist
Saifee Hospital
Mumbai, Maharashtra, India

Rakhi Singh MBBS DGO DRM DPE
FICOG FIAOG
Senior Consultant and IVF Specialist
Obstetrician and Gynecologist
Director of Abalone Clinic and IVF Center
Noida, Uttar Pradesh, India

Rohan Palshetkar MBBS MS (Obs & Gyne)
Consultant
Obstetrics and Gynecology
Palshetkar Patil Nursing Home
Mumbai, Maharashtra, India

Sarita Bhalerao MD DNB FICOG FRCOG
Obstetrician and Gynecologist
Breach Candy, Reliance HN, Saifee
Bhatia and Wadia Maternity Hospitals
Mumbai, Maharashtra, India

Shalini Gainder MD (Obs & Gyne)
DGO FICOG
Gynecologist, Laparoscopic Surgeon
Infertility and IVF Specialist
Postgraduate Institute of Medical
Education and Research
Chandigarh, India

Foreword

It gives me immense pleasure to write foreword for ICOG-Campus, *The Ovary: Recent Developments and Current Practice*.

Ovary is a vital female organ that plays an important role in the reproductive and endocrine system. Changes in lifestyle (Physical inactivity, improper eating habits) and late marriages have led to a lot of reproductive issues. 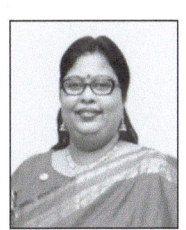 Although all of us manage these conditions in the best possible manner yet time-to-time review helps us keep updated. This book is a comprehensive guide to our current knowledge on physiology of ovarian functions and its disorders and brings out not only salient topics on ovarian disorders but also newer interventions and current concepts in their management.

I appreciate the effort taken by the editor, Dr Madhuri Patil, who has compiled this ICOG Campus of the Ovary.

Wishing you all a very happy new year. May the coming year be more joyous and successful.

S Shantha Kumari
MD DNB FICOG FRCRI (Ireland) FRCOG (UK)
President, FOGSI (2021–22), Treasurer, FIGO (2021–23)
Chairperson, ICOG (2018–19), Secretary, ICOG (2015–17)
Member, FIGO Working Group on
Violence against Women (2015–18)
ICOG Governing Council Member (2012–15)
IAGE Managing Committee Member (2012–18)
National Corresponding Editor for JOGI (2011–13)
Senior Consultant
Department of Obstetrics and Gynecology
Laparoscopic Surgeon
Yashoda Hospitals
Hyderabad, Telangana, India

Foreword

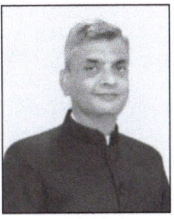

We as practicing gynecologists need to constantly keep ourselves updated on the recent advances in our subject. Ovary is the organ controlling almost all the physiological functions in the woman thought her life. Disorders—PCOS, POF, Endometriosis and Tumors, all are of common occurrence and all have evolving strategies to diagnose and treat. In this Campus, we bring you an overview of the most important topics involving the ovary—from adolescent to menopause.

For this herculean task, we have Dr Madhuri Patil, as an editor, an expert, who goes to the molecular level to explain and treat disorders. I thank her and all the contributors for their efforts to bring out this extremely informative book, and I congratulate Dr Ashok Kumar for accomplishing this task and always being so supportive for all the initiatives taken during my tenure as Chairperson ICOG.

Uday Thanawala
MBBS MD DGO FCPS DNB
Thanawala Maternity Home and IVF Centre
Navi Mumbai, Maharashtra, India
Chairman, ICOG
Treasurer PCOS Society (India)
Vice President, FOGSI (2015)
Chairperson, Medical Disorders
Committee of FOGSI (2006–2008)
Founder Secretary & Past President, NMOGS

Preface

This ICOG Campus on *The Ovary: Recent Developments and Current Practice* deals with the ovarian life cycle. It looks at ovarian function from in-utero to menopause in detail. The chapters represent an unparalleled compilation of relevant to contemporary ovarian physiology and factors related to reproduction, fertility, and menopause. The book has 12 in-depth chapters, which cover different aspects related to the ovary.

The chapter on physiology of ovulation is followed by chapters devoted to ovarian reserve testing, polycystic ovarian syndrome, ovulation induction and its complications, role of adjuvants in ovulation induction and improving ovarian reserve, premature ovarian insufficiency, ovarian aging and its stages and hormonal therapy. All the chapters are well written, logically organized, and easy to read with key messages at the end of each chapter. These chapters will be of great interest to obstetricians–gynecologists.

The book in its current form will be extremely useful for a wide variety of practicing physicians as well as medical students for a quick read to get updates on the subject. I recommend this volume to all those who are interested in women's health and on the topic "Ovary" where several facts are still poorly understood.

Madhuri Patil
Guest Editor, ICOG Campus

Contents

1. **Physiology of Ovulation** 1
   Madhuri Patil

2. **Ovarian Reserve Testing: An Update** 20
   Padma Rekha Jirge

3. **Polycystic Ovarian Syndrome** 28
   Jwal Banker, Duru Shah

4. **Ovulation Induction in Non-assisted Reproductive Technology Cycles** 38
   Chaitanya Shembekar

5. **Can Ovarian Response be Improved in Women with Low Ovarian Reserve?** 50
   Pratik Tambe

6. **Adjuvants in Polycystic Ovary Syndrome** 59
   Rakhi Singh, Meenu Handa, Madhuri Patil

7. **Optimizing Ovarian Stimulation for Assisted Reproductive Technology Outcomes in Women with Advanced Endometriosis** 66
   Shalini Gainder, Parul Kotdawala

8. **Stages of Reproductive Aging and Correlation with Symptoms** 78
   Sarita Bhalerao, Priya Vora

9. **Prevention and Management of Ovarian Hyperstimulation Syndrome** 86
   Fessy Louis T, Meera Ravi Kumar

10. **Premature Ovarian Insufficiency** 97
    Rohan Palshetkar, Nandita Palshetkar, Jiteeka Thakkar

11. **Aging Ovary** 114
    Madhuri Patil, Archana Baser, Anshu Baser

12. **Current Concepts of Hormone Replacement Therapy** 127
    Ashwini Bhalerao Gandhi, Priya Vora, Rajeshwari Khyade

Index *137*

Chapter 1

Physiology of Ovulation

Madhuri Patil

■ INTRODUCTION

Ovulation is a physiologic process by which a mature oocyte is released from a dominant follicle in the ovary into the fallopian tube where it has the potential to fertilize. The application of new forms of research in recent decades has contributed to a more in-depth and accurate understanding of the interaction of each of the inter- and intracellular mechanisms that result in ovulation, implantation, and occurrence of pregnancy. On the other hand, the use of nonhuman primate models has also provided invaluable information in the reproductive field related to ovarian function. Ovulation is under the control of an orchestrated and synchronized secretion of hormones from the hypothalamus, pituitary gland, and ovaries. The major hormones involved are gonadotropin-releasing hormone (GnRH) from the arcuate nucleus of hypothalamus, follicle-stimulating hormone (FSH) and luteinizing hormone (LH) from the pituitary, and estrogen and progesterone (P4) from the ovaries. The normal functioning of the hypothalamic–pituitary–ovarian (HPO) axis is responsible for a normal ovulatory menstrual cycle, which in turn is dependent on a synchronized and pulsatile secretion of the hormones from the hypothalamus and pituitary glands. The secretion of these hormones changes dramatically throughout the menstrual cycle according to the stimulatory or inhibitory signals received from the ovary (secretion of sex steroids) and other autocrine and paracrine factors. The release of the oocyte occurs at the end of the follicular phase (i.e., dominant follicle development) and precedes the luteal phase [i.e., maintenance of corpus luteum (CL)]. This can then result in either a pregnancy if there is fertilization and implantation or endometrial shedding. Ovulation is known to occur usually 14 days prior to menstruation if the HPO axis function is well regulated.

■ OVARIAN RESERVE

Ovarian reserve is the functional potential of the ovary and reflects the number and quality of oocytes within it. Thus, it is the capacity of the ovaries to provide oocytes that are capable of fertilization resulting in a healthy and successful pregnancy. The quantity of oocytes depends on ovarian age, whereas the quality of oocytes depends on chronological age.

The female fetus has maximum oogonia at the gestational age of 20 weeks. Thereafter, the number of oocytes decreases and at birth there are only 2–3 million and at menarche there would be only 3,00,000–4,00,000 left. Thus, the female has lost most of her oocytes till she reaches her reproductive age. Over her entire reproductive life span, only about 400 oocytes would have grown and ovulated. Thus, depletion of oocytes begins before birth, and continues until menopause. The rate of this depletion is fairly constant over a woman's lifespan but accelerates at around the age of 37 years. At the beginning of every menstrual cycle, a fixed proportion of all remaining oocytes acquires gonadotropin (GT) sensitivity. These oocytes are selected 3 months prior to the cycle in which they are destined to grow and ovulate or undergo apoptosis. In a natural cycle, all but one of these recruitable oocytes in the follicle undergo atresia, which correlates with the woman's age. The size of the cohort of recruitable follicles is much larger in the younger women as compared to the older women.

Prior to menopause, there is subtle elevation in the FSH and decrease in inhibin B concentration, which makes the menstrual cycles shorter. This is seen on ultrasound as small ovaries with fewer antral follicles on day 2 of the cycle. The decreased ovarian reserve results in ovulation of fewer eggs, which may have a compromised quality and thus there is occurrence of fewer pregnancy with increase in miscarriage rate and decrease in live birth rate.

Thus, ovarian reserve tells us about:
- Oocytes within the ovaries
- Growing follicles
- Small antral follicles
- Follicles that can be stimulated by FSH
- Oocytes that can be recovered after FSH.

Ovarian reserve tests provide information about the size of the antral follicle cohort, which is proportionally related to the primordial follicle pool. None of these tests tells us about the occurrence of pregnancy. **Flowchart 1** enumerates the various ovarian tests available.

Today, the ovarian reserve is assessed by measuring the anti-Müllerian hormone (AMH) and evaluating the antral follicle count (AFC) by ultrasound. Apart from this, age is an important predictor of ovarian reserve and fertility. Female fertility declines with age, which is both quantitative and qualitative;[1] however, age per se can be a poor determinant of female fertility, since there is a wide range of variation in the relationship between ovarian reserve and age.[2] FSH is no longer used as an ovarian reserve test as it does not diagnose poor ovarian reserve until high thresholds are reached,[3] and it also has extreme inter- and intracycle variations that limit its reliability.[4] Moreover, elevated

Physiology of Ovulation

Flowchart 1: Ovarian reserve tests (ORT).

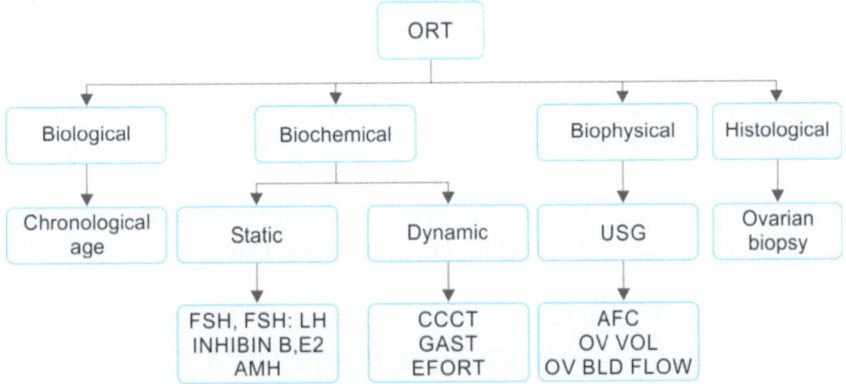

(AFC: antral follicle count; AMH: anti-Müllerian hormone; CCCT: clomiphene citrate challenge test; E2: estradiol; EFORT: exogenous follicle-stimulating hormone ovarian reserve test; FSH: follicle-stimulating hormone; GAST: gonadotropin-releasing hormone agonist stimulation test; LH: luteinizing hormone; OV BLD: ovarian blood; OV VOL: ovarian volume; USG: ultrasonography)

day 3 FSH is a heterogeneous group, which might suggest a true reduced ovarian reserve or may be due to the presence of heterophilic antibodies or FSH receptor polymorphism in patients with otherwise normal ovaries.[5]

■ PHYSIOLOGY OF MENSTRUAL CYCLE

Menstruation is defined as periodic and cyclic shedding of endometrium accompanied by loss of blood. There are three phases of menstrual cycle:
1. Follicular phase—recruitment and growth of a cohort of follicles that result in the formation of single mature follicle
2. Ovulatory phase—final maturation and release of oocyte
3. Luteal phase—formation of CL to secrete hormones to support implantation.

Gonadotropin-releasing hormone secreted by hypothalamus via neural mechanisms controls the pituitary–gonadal axis, which requires presence of remarkable coordination of hormonal secretions and morphological and cellular changes at various levels. Hypothalamic GnRH is a neurohormone, a decapeptide, which is released in a pulsatile manner every 1–2 hours and plays an important role in the neurohormonal control of the hypothalamic–pituitary–gonadal axis. It controls the secretion of FSH and LH from the pituitary, which in turn results in folliculogenesis with growth of the primordial follicles and production and secretion of gonadal steroids, estrogen, and P4. Disturbed pulses are seen in stress, exercise, and nutrition, which can result in prolonged follicular phase, luteal phase deficiency (LPD), anovulation, and amenorrhea. Synthesis and release of GT from the pituitary is regulated by release of an array of second messengers and the activation of several intracellular pathways that result from the interaction of GnRH with specific G-protein-coupled receptors located on the surface of gonadotrophs.

These include the activation of phospholipase C with the ensuing production of diacylglycerol and inositol-trisphosphate, which are responsible for the activation of protein kinase C and the mobilization of intracellular Ca^{2+}, respectively. Activation of phospholipases D and A2, and production of cyclic adenosine monophosphate (cAMP) and cyclic guanosine monophosphate (cGMP) occur in response to GnRH. GnRH also results in the activation of tyrosine kinases and the mitogen-activated protein (MAP) kinase cascade in certain circumstances. Evidence suggests the presence of extrapituitary receptors, which respond to locally produced GnRH (in gonads, placenta, mammary gland, etc.). *Pituitary gonadotrophs*: FSH and LH have similar α subunits but different β subunits. Both are released rapidly in response to GnRH and act on granulosa, theca, and luteal cells in ovaries to secrete estrogen (E2) and P4. The amount of estrogen and P4 secreted depends on the stage of the follicular development, and this in turn through its positive and negative feedback mechanism will control the secretion of FSH and LH. Thus, the secretion of FSH and LH in turn depends on the stage of the follicular development.

Although all follicles have equal potential to reach full maturation, only follicles that have a lower threshold and competent oocyte during the rise in FSH in the follicular phase will gain GT dependence. The FSH concentration above which the follicles develop GT dependence is called the FSH threshold.[6] Follicles respond to exogenous administration of FSH only if the FSH concentrations rise above the FSH threshold. The other factors that affect the response of the ovary to FSH include woman's age, body mass index (BMI), AFC, inhibin B, AMH, and growth factors.[7] The folliculogenesis and ovulation of a mature oocyte can also be affected by the presence of other endocrinological conditions such as hyperprolactinemia, polycystic ovarian syndrome (PCOS), and adrenal hyperandrogenemia.[7]

Functions of FSH:
- Recruitment of antral follicles
- Selection and maturation of dominant follicle
- Granulosa cell differentiation and growth
- Activation of aromatase enzyme system resulting in E2 secretion
- FSH receptor increase on granulosa cells
- Induction of LH receptors on granulosa cells
- Production of autocrine–paracrine factors, especially activin and inhibin.

Functions of LH: These functions are different in different phases of menstrual cycle:
- *Follicular phase:*
  - Promotes androgen secretion in theca

- Synergic action with FSH in producing E2
- Support dominance once FSH levels
- *Midcycle phase:*
  - Resumption of oocyte meiosis
  - Maturation of cumulus–oocyte complex (COC)
  - Follicular rupture
  - Granulosa luteinization
- *Luteal phase:*
  - Maintenance of CL and P4 secretion
  - Induces endometrial receptivity for implantation.

■ PITUITARY OVARIAN CYCLE (FIG. 1)

A critical range of pulsatile GnRH secretion (frequency and amplitude) is necessary for normal reproductive function. Synthesis, storage, activation, and secretion of FSH and LH are a result of positive action of GnRH on the anterior pituitary. The GT are also secreted in a pulsatile fashion in response to the pulsatile release of GnRH from the hypothalamus. Lower GnRH pulse frequencies favor FSH secretion, while higher GnRH pulse frequencies favor LH secretion. Apart from GnRH, the secretion of FSH and LH is also governed by steroids (estrogen and P4) secreted in the ovaries as a result of folliculogenesis, activin, inhibin, and follistatin produced in response to FSH.

Low levels of estrogen enhance FSH and LH synthesis and storage, and result in the secretion of FSH to stimulate folliculogenesis. As follicles grow, the amount of estrogen secretion increases, which selectively decreases the secretion of FSH. High levels of estrogen from a dominant follicle are responsible for the induction of mid-cyclic LH surge. When estrogen levels are maintained high during this period, it results in a corresponding sustained elevated LH secretion. A small rise in P4 level just before the LH surge enhances the LH response to GnRH at the pituitary level and is also responsible for the FSH surge at midcycle. Pituitary secretion of GT is inhibited by the high levels of P4 in the luteal phase, which inhibit the GnRH secretion at the level of the hypothalamus. High levels of P4 also antagonize pituitary response to GnRH by interfering with estrogen action. The synthesis and secretion of pituitary GT are also influenced to varying degrees, by activin, inhibin, and follistatin apart from hypothalamic GnRH.[8] Activin enhances and follistatin suppresses GnRH activity. Prolonged GnRH stimulation results in downregulation of pituitary GT secretion as continuous GnRH stimulation increases the follistatin production, which then blocks the GT response to GnRH stimulation. As the follicle grows, the follistatin level increases and activin decreases.[8] Inhibin B production is enhanced by FSH and estradiol in the early follicular phase, whereas in the late follicular

Physiology of Ovulation

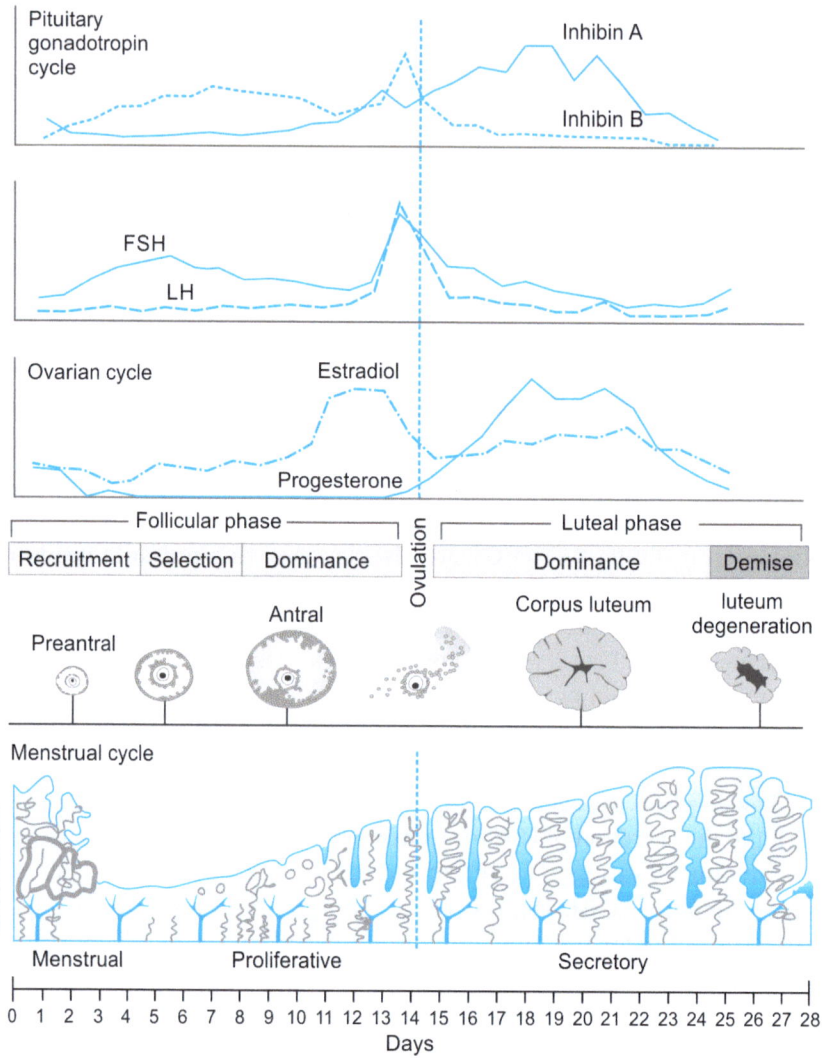

Fig. 1: Pituitary, ovarian, and menstrual cycle. (FSH: follicle-stimulating hormone; LH: luteinizing hormone)

phase, the secretion of inhibin A increases as a result of increase in LH levels. Increased levels of inhibin B and decreased levels of activin in the late follicular phase promote androgen synthesis in the theca cells in response to LH and insulin-like growth factor II (IGF-II). This androgen produced acts as a substrate for increased estrogen production in the granulosa cells of the dominant follicle. LH secretion, on the other hand, is not influenced by inhibin–activin–follistatin system and is primarily regulated by GnRH.

The changes in the ovarian hormonal levels are reflected in the endometrium, which is proliferative in the follicular phase and secretory in the luteal phase (**Fig. 1**). Menstruation occurs in the luteal–follicular transition phase due to the demise of the CL, which results in a nadir in the circulating levels of estradiol, P4, and inhibin. The decrease in inhibin A removes a suppressing influence on FSH secretion in the pituitary, while decrease in estradiol and P4 allows a progressive and rapid increase in the frequency of GnRH pulsatile secretion and a removal of the pituitary from negative feedback suppression. Increase in GnRH pulse frequency from the luteal phase frequency of every 4 hours to follicular phase frequency of every 90 minutes is essential to recreate the normal intercycle rise in FSH. The removal of inhibin A and estradiol and increasing GnRH pulses combine to allow greater secretion of FSH compared with LH, with an increase in the frequency of the episodic secretion. The increase in FSH is instrumental in rescuing approximately a 70-day-old group of ready follicles from atresia, allowing a dominant follicle to begin its emergence.

FOLLICULAR RECRUITMENT AND GROWTH IN A NATURAL MENSTRUAL CYCLE

Follicle development (**Fig. 2**) from the primordial to the preovulatory stage takes several months.[9] The initiation of growth of the primordial follicles takes place continuously throughout the female life and is under paracrine control and independent of pituitary GT. This selection usually occurs 90–120 days before the cycle in which they are destined to ovulate.

The mechanism for determining which follicles and how many will start growing during any one cycle is unknown. But it has been observed that the

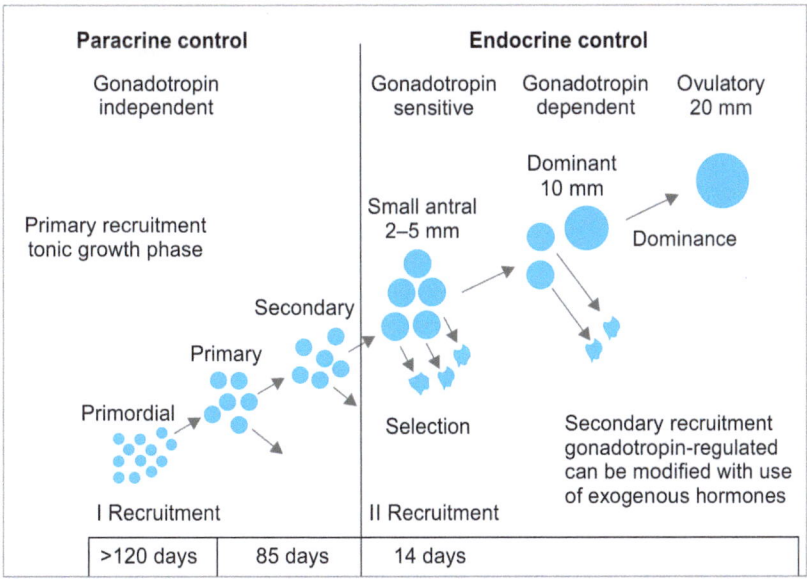

Fig. 2: Selection of dominant follicle.

number of follicles that starts growing each cycle is dependent on the ovarian reserve, which in turn depends on the number of primordial follicles.[10,11]

The activation of primordial follicles is a complex but orchestrated process, which is regulated by multiple factors and pathways. The phosphoinositide 3-kinase (PI3K)–serine/threonine protein kinase (Akt)–forkhead box O3 (FOXO3) signaling pathway plays a key role in the maintenance of primordial follicles, while the mammalian target of rapamycin (mTOR) signal regulates the activation of primordial follicles.[12] Pattern of signaling of KL/c-Kit system via PI3K-Akt-FKHRL1 and phosphatase and tensin homolog (PTEN) is illustrated in **Flowchart 2**. Factors such as FOXL2, Sohlh1, NOBOX, GDF-9, BMP4, BMP7, bFGF, and EGF initiate the activation of primordial follicles, whereas Lhx8 and AMH are suppressive factors in this process.[13]

Thus, inhibition of PTEN results in PI3K activation, which then results in follicle recruitment. GDF-9 and BMP-15 act through direct physical contact at the granulosa cell–oocyte interface, which then modifies the proliferation, function, and differentiation of granulosa cells and activates the oocyte to grow.[14-16]

Flowchart 2: Phosphoinositide 3-kinase (PI3K)–serine/threonine protein kinase (Akt)–forkhead box O3 (FOXO3) signaling pathway.

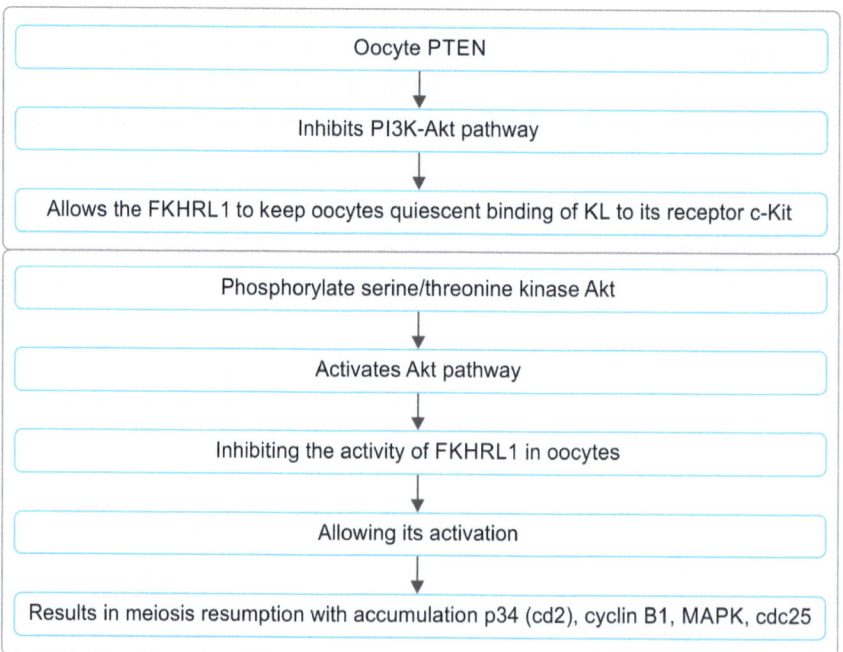

(Akt: protein kinase B (PKB); KL; Kit ligand; c-Kit: receptor tyrosine kinase; FOXO: 3A or FKHRL-1-Forkhead1; MAPK: mitogen-activated protein kinases; p34: protein kinase; Cyclin B: regulatory subunit of M-phase promoting factor; cdc25: cell division cycle 25; PI3K: phosphoinositide 3-kinase; PTEN: phosphatase and tensin homolog)

Once activated to grow, oocytes orchestrate and coordinate the development of ovarian follicles. Thus, the rate of follicle development is controlled by oocyte itself. Appropriate levels of GT, particularly FSH, are required for the development of preantral follicle to antral follicle and then into a preovulatory one. FSH during the follicular phase increases estrogen production from the follicle and then estrogen and FSH act synergistically to increase the FSH receptor content of the growing follicle and also induce the formation of LH receptors on the granulosa cells once the dominance of the follicle is achieved. Early antral follicles thus have only FSH receptors on the granulosa cells and therefore are FSH responsive **(Fig. 2)**. FSH stimulates the growth of the follicle in the early follicular phase. In the late follicular phase, once the LH receptors are induced on the granulosa cells, the follicle becomes responsive to both FSH and LH.[17] Therefore, it is important to understand the two-cell, two-gonadotropin theory **(Fig. 3)**.

The two-cell, two-gonadotropin theory gives information on follicular development and steroidogenesis. The follicular phase of the menstrual cycle accounts for the last 2 weeks of follicle development, which involves growth and maturation of the follicle. The growth and steroidogenesis are dependent on FSH and LH secreted by the pituitary.[18] Follicular selection is achieved from mid-follicular through late-follicular phase. During folliculogenesis, the granulosa cells acquire aromatase activity. This increase in aromatase activity

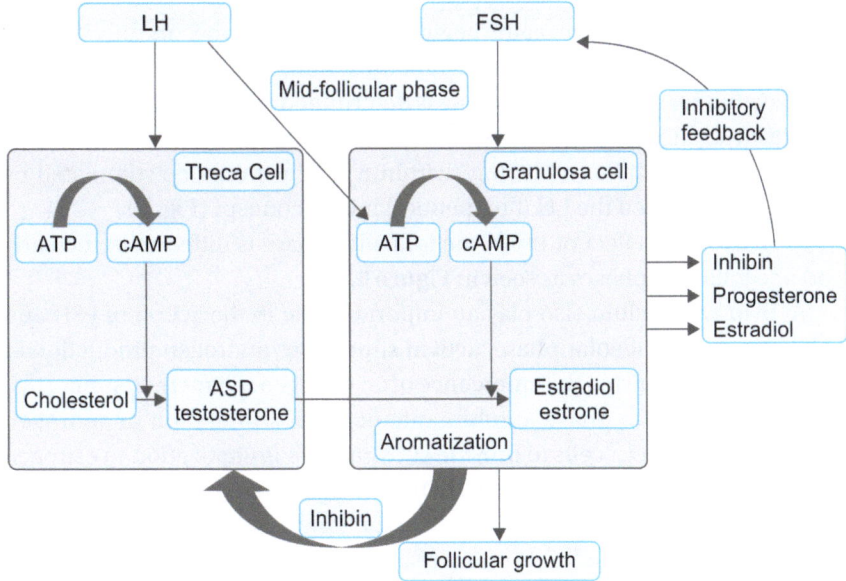

Fig. 3: Two-cell, two-gonadotropin theory. (ASD: androstenedione; ATP: adenosine triphosphate; cAMP: cyclic adenosine monophosphate; FSH: follicle-stimulating hormone; LH: luteinizing hormone)

increases the estradiol and inhibin levels with consequent progressive fall in FSH serum concentration due to negative feedback. This mid-follicular fall in FSH concentration results in atresia of less mature follicles that are unable to grow without adequate FSH concentrations.[18] Apart from increase in aromatase activity, mid-follicular phase FSH also increases the number of FSH and LH receptors in the granulosa cell of the dominant follicle, which can then utilize LH for its further growth and maturation despite the falling FSH levels. LH will increase the androgen production in theca cells, which diffuses into the granulosa cells, where it will be converted to estradiol by the aromatase enzyme.

The action of LH on its receptors in the granulosa cells activates adenyl cyclase with consequent production of cAMP.[19] With this, the maturing follicle reduces its dependency on FSH by acquiring LH receptors and LH responsiveness and continues to grow until final maturation to the preovulatory stage with subsequent ovulation.[20]

Thus, the two-cell, two-gonadotropins theory suggests that LH not only has a role in steroidogenesis in the theca cells but is also involved in follicular growth and maturation in the late follicular phase. FSH, on the other hand, controls the major morphological cellular events in the follicle and is a principal regulator of follicular growth. LH negatively regulates cell growth while positively regulating steroid synthesis.[18]

■ THRESHOLD CONCEPT[21,22]

- Follicular development at the beginning of each cycle occurs only if serum FSH concentration exceeds a certain threshold.
- The number of follicles to ovulate is determined by the length of time that the level of FSH remains above the threshold value.
- The follicle also has a "ceiling" within which it should be stimulated by LH. This is called the LH therapeutic window concept **(Fig. 4)**.

Moreover, the effect of LH in the follicular phase is different in the early and late follicular phases as seen in **Figure 5**.[23]

Activin and inhibin also play an important role in the action of FSH and LH. In the early follicular phase, activin suppresses androgen production in the theca cells, allowing the emergence of an estrogen microenvironment.[24-26] In the late follicular phase, inhibin enhances LH stimulation of androgen synthesis in the theca cells to provide substrate for aromatization to estrogen in the granulosa cells. The increase in the estrogen apart from its feedback to the hypothalamus and pituitary is necessary for local follicular actions and to trigger the LH surge.[24-26] With increasing levels of estrogen, inhibin B is secreted by the granulosa cells into the circulation. Increasing levels of both E2 and inhibin B decrease FSH secretion, and this insufficient FSH is unable to keep smaller follicles growing, which then become atretic and undergo

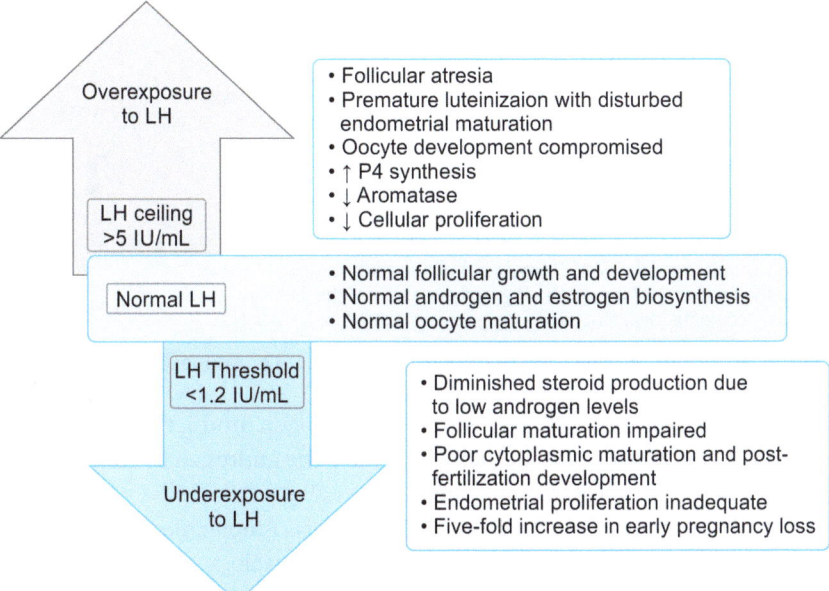

Fig. 4: Luteinizing hormone (LH) therapeutic window concept. (P4: progesterone)

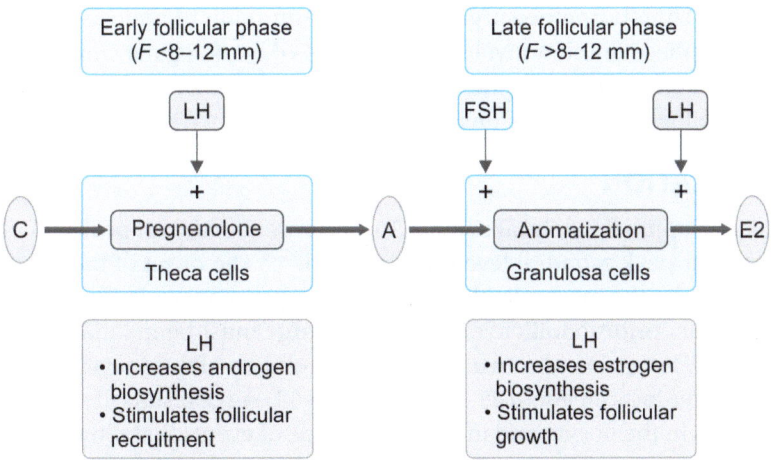

Fig. 5: Effect of luteinizing hormone (LH) in follicular phase. (E2: estradiol; FSH: follicle-stimulating hormone)

apoptosis. Only the dominant follicle with maximum receptors for both FSH and LH can utilize the FSH and LH and survives to grow further and ovulate.

Thus, the events in the mid-follicular phase can be summarized as follows:
- Mid-follicular rise in E2 exerts negative feedback on hypothalamus with decrease in FSH and positive feedback effect on LH.

Flowchart 3: Events in preovulatory follicle.

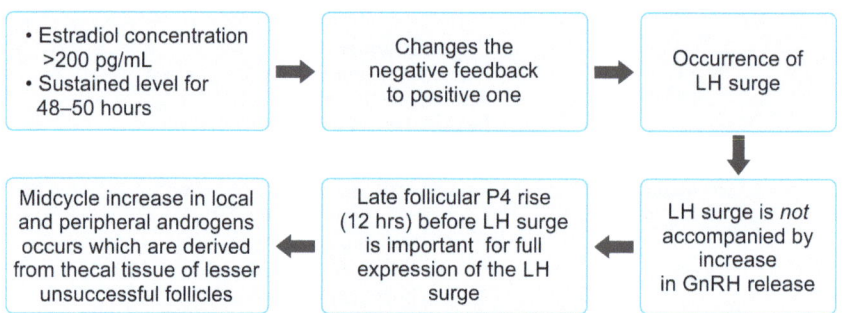

(GnRH: gonadotropin-releasing hormone; LH: luteinizing hormone; P4: progesterone)

- Late follicular high LH levels stimulate androgen production in the theca, and FSH allows dominant follicle to utilize the androgen as substrate and further accelerate estrogen production.
- Positive action of E2 includes modification of GT molecule with increasing bioactivity and quantity of FSH and LH at midcycle.
- P4 reduces GnRH pulse frequency in E2 primed environment.

The events in preovulatory follicles with the onset of LH surge are shown in **Flowchart 3**.

Luteinizing hormone surge results in resumption of meiosis where the first metaphase division involves segregation of homologous chromosomes from each other and metaphase II involves segregation of sister chromatids that is analogous to mitotic division.

OVULATION

Ovulation approximately takes place 10–12 hours after the LH peak and 24–36 hours after peak estradiol levels are attained.[27,28] The onset of the LH surge appears to be the most reliable indicator of impending ovulation, occurring 34–36 hours prior to follicle rupture.[29] LH surge must be maintained for at least 14–27 hours in order to achieve full maturation of the oocyte.[30] Usually, the LH surge lasts for about 48–50 hours.[29] The LH surge results in resumption of meiosis in the oocyte and initiates a cascade of events that ultimately lead to ovulation. Ovulation involves the physical release of the oocyte, and its cumulus mass of granulosa cells.[31] The final meiotic division is not completed until the sperm has entered the oocyte resulting in fertilization and extrusion of the second polar body.

With the LH surge, levels of P4 rise till the time of ovulation. This rise in P4 has a negative feedback effect and terminates the LH surge. P4 also increases the distensibility of the follicle wall. Mid-cyclic rise in FSH, LH, and P4 stimulates the activity of proteolytic enzymes, resulting in digestion of collagen in the follicular wall and increasing its distensibility followed by release of the ovum.

■ LUTEAL PHASE

Ovulation is followed by luteal phase, which is defined as the period from occurrence of ovulation until the establishment of a pregnancy or the resumption of menses 2 weeks later. Luteal phase reflects the functional life span of the CL, which is a temporary endocrine gland. *Lifespan:* 14 ± 2 days and is formed from the remnants of the ruptured follicle. It is a major source of steroid hormones and secretes up to 40 mg of P4 per day. In the luteal phase, the three hormones that are crucial are:

1. P4
2. Estradiol
3. LH.

The role of LH is the most crucial and is totally responsible for steroidogenic activity of the CL,[32] upregulation of growth factors, vascular endothelial growth factor A (VEGF-A), fibroblast growth factor 2 (FGF2), and cytokines involved in implantation[33,34] and stimulation of LH receptors in endometrium.[35]

Luteal P4 rise is important and plays a critical role in implantation and development of normal pregnancy by the following:

- Downregulating the number of estrogen receptors (ERs), thus indirectly suppressing the inhibitory effects of E2 on integrins
- Acts positively by increasing paracrine stromal factors—EGF and heparin-binding EGF (HB-EGF)[36]
- Direct effect by stimulating homeobox gene *HOXA 10*—implicated in the regulation of β3 subunit expression.[37]

■ LUTEAL–FOLLICULAR TRANSITION

At the end of the luteal phase, small antral follicles (2–5 mm in diameter) are present and the granulosa cells of these are more sensitive to FSH stimulation. During the luteofollicular transition, demise of the CL results in decreased production of both estrogen and P4. This decrease results in the negative feedback effect with increase in the FSH serum concentration (perimenstrual rise). This rise in FSH in the early follicular phase maintains a plateau and must reach a threshold to result in recruitment of a new ovulating follicle, which has a low FSH threshold. Thus, a critical concentration of FSH must be achieved to initiate the process of follicular development in the menstrual cycle.[38-41]

■ ROLE OF NEUROKININ B/DYNORPHIN/KISSPEPTIN

Neuropeptides, kisspeptin, neurokinin B, and dynorphin (KNDy) play a key role in the physiological regulation of GnRH neurons.[42] Kiss1 neurons in the arcuate nucleus is a plausible generator of GnRH pulses through a system of pulsatile kisspeptin release, which is influenced by a coordinated action of neurokinin B (NKB) and dynorphin (DYN) A.[43] Neuroendocrine defects seen in clinical reproductive disorders such as PCOS may be related to alterations in KNDy cell peptide.

- NKB has a role in steroid feedback control of GnRH release.
- DYN is an endogenous opioid peptide, which acts primarily through the κ-opioid receptor (KOR) and is known to regulate P4-mediated negative feedback on GnRH release, thus inhibiting GnRH secretion.
- Kisspeptin acts together with NKB and DYN in a complex manner to precisely regulate GnRH pulse generation in response to dynamic changes in steroid hormone concentrations. Kisspeptin, apart from stimulation of GnRH secretion, mediates negative and positive feedback effects of sex steroids on the hypothalamus.[42] Kisspeptin expression in the ovary mainly occurs in the granulosa cells in response to preovulatory LH surge. Its signaling drives oocyte survival through the PI3K/Akt pathway. It also stimulates steroid secretion by theca and luteal cells.

Hormonal changes during folliculogenesis are reflected as endometrial changes. Thus, endometrial thickness and morphology are a reliable bioassay of the patient's hormonal status and changes correlate with plasma estrogen and P4 levels. In the follicular phase, estrogen results in proliferation, and thickening of the mucosa with increasing cell numbers and size. This is seen as translucent and thin on either side of midline echo in the early follicular phase followed by increase in thickness with a hyporeflective area in the center in the late follicular phase. In the luteal phase, the endometrium shrinks in thickness, and is dense echogenic on either side of midline echo.

■ CONCLUSION

Ovulation involves perfect synchronization between neuronal, hormonal, and local events.

Ovarian follicle development is regulated by the HPO axis, in which GnRH controls the release of the gonadotropic hormones FSH and LH, and ovarian steroids exert both negative and positive regulatory effects on GnRH secretion. Other intraovarian signaling cascades affect follicular development and GT action in a stage- and context-specific manner. Endometrial preparation follows a well-documented pattern—growth in the first phase and decidualization in the second phase. Any disturbance in the events leading to midcycle surge and luteal phase can disrupt the local changes within the endometrium and hence affect implantation. Endocrine mechanisms ensure monofollicular development in a menstrual cycle, and manipulations of these mechanisms are used for ovulation induction and superovulation.

Physiology of Ovulation

KEY MESSAGES

- *Neuroendocrine control of reproduction requires:*

  Pulsatile secretion of GnRH is released into the pituitary portal system
  ↓
  Stimulates the synthesis and secretion of LH and FSH from the gonadotrophs
  ↓
  GT FSH and LH, in turn, stimulate follicular development and secretion of gonadal steroids and peptides
  ↓
  Which have negative feedback effects on the hypothalamus and pituitary resulting in decreased FSH secretion
  ↓
  At midcycle, rising levels of E2 are responsible for the positive feedback that results in the preovulatory LH surge

- *Key points in regulation of HPO axis:*
  - For normal reproductive function, it is absolutely necessary for the pulsatile GnRH secretion to be within a critical range with adequate frequency, concentration, and amplitude.
  - GnRH has only positive actions on the anterior pituitary resulting in synthesis, storage, activation, and secretion of FSH and LH.
  - GT FSH and LH are secreted in a pulsatile fashion in response to the similar pulsatile release of GnRH.
  - Lower GnRH pulse frequencies favor FSH secretion, and higher GnRH pulse frequencies favor LH secretion.
  - Low levels of estrogen enhance FSH and LH synthesis and storage.
  - Estrogen has little effect on LH secretion but inhibits FSH secretion.
  - High levels of estrogen induce the mid-cyclic LH surge.
  - Low levels of P4 acting at the level of the pituitary gland enhance the LH response to GnRH and are responsible for FSH surge at midcycle.
  - High levels of P4 inhibit pituitary secretion of GTs by inhibiting GnRH pulses at the level of the hypothalamus.
  - High levels of P4 can also antagonize pituitary response to GnRH by interfering with estrogen action.

- *Events in antral follicle:*
  - Mid-follicular rise in E2 exerts negative feedback on hypothalamus with decrease in FSH.
  - Late follicular rise in estrogen has a positive feedback effect on LH secretion.
  - Late follicular high LH levels stimulate androgen production in the theca and FSH allows dominant follicle to utilize the androgen as substrate and further accelerate estrogen production.
  - Positive action of E2 includes modification of GT molecule with increasing bioactivity and quantity of both FSH and LH at midcycle.
  - P4 reduces GnRH pulse frequency in E2 primed environment.

- *Event in preovulatory follicles—LH surge:*
  - Estrogen production becomes sufficient to achieve and maintain peripheral threshold concentrations of estradiol that are required in order to induce the LH surge.

Contd...

Contd…

- Acting through its receptors, LH initiates luteinization and P4 production in the granulosa layer.
- The preovulatory rise in P4 facilitates the positive feedback action of estrogen and may be required to induce the midcycle FSH peak.
- A midcycle increase in local and peripheral androgens occurs, derived from the theca tissue of lesser, unsuccessful follicles.

- *Key ovulatory events are as follows:*
  - LH surge also stimulates luteinization of granulosa cells and synthesis of P4 and prostaglandin (PG) within the follicle.
  - P4 enhances the activity of proteolytic enzymes and together with PG is responsible for digestion and rupture of follicular wall.
  - *P4 also results in midcycle rise in FSH*:
    - Is important to free the oocyte from follicular attachments
    - To convert plasminogen to proteolytic enzymes plasmin
    - To ensure that sufficient LH receptors are present to allow adequate normal luteal phase
  - Final meiotic division occurs only after fertilization.

- *Events in the luteal phase:*
  - Normal luteal function requires optimal preovulatory follicular development and continued tonic LH support.
  - P4 acts both centrally and within the ovary to suppress new follicular growth.
  - Regression of CL may involve luteolytic action with decrease in both estrogen and P4 production, which is mediated by alteration in local PG and endothelin 1 concentrations.
  - If pregnancy occurs, human chorionic gonadotropin (hCG) rescues the CL, maintaining its function until placental steroidogenesis is well established.

- *Events in luteal–follicular transition:*
  - Demise of CL results in decreasing circulating levels of E2, P4, and inhibin.
  - Decrease in inhibin A removes its suppressive effect on FSH secretion in the pituitary.
  - Decrease in E2 and P4 allows progressive and rapid increase in frequency of GnRH pulsatile secretion and removal of pituitary from negative feedback suppression.
  - Combined effect of removal of inhibin A and E2 and increasing GnRH pulses allows greater secretion of FSH compared to LH.
  - Increase in FSH is instrumental in rescuing approximately 60-day-old group of small antral follicles from atresia and allowing emergence of a dominant follicle.

REFERENCES

1. te Velde ER, Pearson PL. The variability of female reproductive ageing. Hum Reprod Update. 2002;8(2):141-54.
2. Maroulis GB. Effect of aging on fertility and pregnancy. Semin Reprod Endocrinol. 1991;9(3):165-75.
3. van Rooij IA, Bancsi LF, Broekmans FJ, Looman CW, Habbema JD, te Velde ER. Women older than 40 years of age and those with elevated follicle-stimulating hormone levels differ in poor response rate and embryo quality in in vitro fertilization. Fertil Steril. 2003;79(3):482-8.

4. Kwee J, Schats R, McDonnell J, Lambalk CB, Schoemaker J. Intercycle variability of ovarian reserve tests: results of a prospective randomized study. Hum Reprod. 2004;19:590-5.
5. Lambalk CB. Value of elevated basal follicle-stimulating hormone levels and the differential diagnosis during the diagnostic subfertility work-up. Fertil Steril. 2003;79(3):489-90.
6. Brown JB. Pituitary control of ovarian function—concepts derived from gonadotrophin therapy. Aust N Z J Obstet Gynaecol. 1978;18(1):47-54.
7. Fauser BC, van Heusden AM. Manipulation of human ovarian function: physiological concepts and clinical consequences. Endocr Rev. 1997;18(1):71-106.
8. de Kretser DM, Hedger MP, Loveland KL, Phillips DJ. Inhibins, activins and follistatin in reproduction. Hum Reprod Update. 2002;8(6):529-41.
9. Gougeon A. Regulation of ovarian follicular development in primates: facts and hypotheses. Endocr Rev. 1996;17:121.
10. Peters H, Byskov AG, Himelstein-Graw R, Faber M. Follicular growth: the basic event in the mouse and human ovary. J Reprod Fertil. 1975;45:559.
11. Gougeon A, Echochard R, Thalabard JC. Age-related changes of the population of human ovarian follicles: increase in the disappearance rate of non-growing and early-growing follicles in aging women. Biol Reprod. 1994;50:653.
12. Artini PG, Tatone C, Sperduti S, D'Aurora M, Franchi S, Di Emidio G, et al. Cumulus cells surrounding oocytes with high developmental competence exhibit down-regulation of phosphoinositol 1,3 kinase/protein kinase B (PI3K/AKT) signalling genes involved in proliferation and survival. Hum Reprod. 2017;32(12):2474-84.
13. Li L, Shi X, Shi Y, Wang Z. The signaling pathways involved in ovarian follicle development. Front Physiol. 2021;12:730196.
14. Yan C, Wang P, De Mayo J, De Mayo FJ, Elvin JA, Carino C, et al. Synergistic roles of bone morphogenetic protein 15 and growth differentiation factor 9 in ovarian function. Mol Endocrinol. 2001;15(6):854-66.
15. Moore RK, Erickson GF, Shimasaki S. Are BMP-15 and GDF-9 primary determinants of ovulation quota in mammals? Trends Endocrinol Metab. 2004;15(8):356-61.
16. McMahon HE, Sharma S, Shimasaki S. Phosphorylation of bone morphogenetic protein-15 and growth and differentiation factor-9 plays a critical role in determining agonistic or antagonistic functions. Endocrinology. 2008;149(2):812-7.
17. Zeleznik AJ, Hillier SG. The role of gonadotropins in the selection of the preovulatory follicle. Clin Obstet Gynecol. 1984;27:927.
18. Hillier SG. Current concepts of the roles of follicle stimulating hormone and luteinizing hormone in folliculogenesis. Hum Reprod. 1994;9(2):188-91.
19. Goff AK, Armstrong DT. Stimulatory action of gonadotropins and prostaglandins on adenosine-3',5'-monophosphate production by isolated rat granulosa cells. Endocrinology. 1977;101(5):1461-7.
20. Filicori M, Cognigni GE, Tabarelli C, Pocognoli P, Taraborrelli S, Spettoli D, et al. Stimulation and growth of antral ovarian follicles by selective LH activity administration in women. J Clin Endocrinol Metab. 2002;87:1156.
21. Schipper I, Hop WC, Fauser BC. The follicle-stimulating hormone (FSH) threshold/window concept examined by different interventions with exogenous

FSH during the follicular phase of the normal menstrual cycle: duration, rather than magnitude, of FSH increase affects follicle development. J Clin Endocrinol Metab. 1998;83(4):1292-8.
22. Palermo R. Differential actions of FSH and LH during folliculogenesis. Reprod Biomed Online. 2007;15(3):326-37.
23. de Ziegler D, Fraisse T, de Candolle G, Vulliemoz N, Bellavia M, Colamaria S. Roles of FSH and LH during the follicular phase: insight into natural cycle IVF. Reprod Biomed Online. 2007;15(5):507-13.
24. Lockwood GM, Muttukrishna S, Ledger WL. Inhibins and activins in human ovulation, conception and pregnancy. Hum Reprod Update. 1998;4(3):284-95.
25. Namwanje M, Brown CW. Activins and inhibins: roles in development, physiology, and disease. Cold Spring Harb Perspect Biol. 2016;8(7):a021881.
26. Adu-Gyamfi EA, Djankpa FT, Nelson W, Czika A, Sah SK, Lamptey J, et al. Activin and inhibin signaling: from regulation of physiology to involvement in the pathology of the female reproductive system. Cytokine. 2020;133:155105.
27. Pauerstein CJ, Eddy CA, Croxatto HD, Hess R, Siler-Khodr TM, Croxatto HB. Temporal relationships of estrogen, progesterone, and luteinizing hormone levels to ovulation in women and infrahuman primates. Am J Obstet Gynecol. 1978;130:876.
28. World Health Organization, Task Force on Methods for the Determination of the Fertile Period, Special Programme of Research, Development and Research Training in Human Reproduction. Temporal relationships between ovulation and defined changes in the concentration of plasma estradiol-17β, luteinizing hormone, follicle stimulating hormone, and progesterone. I. Probit analysis. Am J Obstet Gynecol. 1980;138:383-90.
29. Hoff JD, Quigley ME, Yen SS. Hormonal dynamics at midcycle: a reevaluation. J Clin Endocrinol Metab. 1983;57:792.
30. Zelinski-Wooten MB, Hutchison JS, Chandrasekher YA, Wolf DP, Stouffer RL. Administration of human luteinizing hormone (hLH) to Macaques after follicular development: further titration of LH surge requirements for ovulatory changes in primate follicles. J Clin Endocrinol Metab. 1992;75:502.
31. Yoshimura Y, Wallach EE. Studies on the mechanism(s) of mammalian ovulation. Fertil Steril. 1987;47:22.
32. Casper RF, Yen SS, Wilkes MM. Menopausal flushes: a neuroendocrine link with pulsatile luteinizing hormone secretion. Science. 1979;205(4408):823-5.
33. Sugino N, Karube-Harada A, Taketani T, Sakata A, Nakamura Y. Withdrawal of ovarian steroids stimulates prostaglandin F2α production through nuclear factor-κB activation via oxygen radicals in human endometrial stromal cells: potential relevance to menstruation. J Reprod Dev. 2004;50(2):215-25.
34. Licht P, Russu V, Wildt L. On the role of human chorionic gonadotropin (hCG) in the embryo-endometrial microenvironment: implications for differentiation and implantation. Semin Reprod Med. 2001;19(1):37-48.
35. Tesarik J, Hazout A, Mendoza C. Luteinizing hormone affects uterine receptivity independently of ovarian function. Reprod Biomed Online. 2003;7(1):59-64.
36. Achache H, Revel A. Endometrial receptivity markers, the journey to successful embryo implantation. Hum Reprod Update. 2006;12(6):731-46.
37. Lessey BA. Two pathways of progesterone action in the human endometrium: implications for implantation and contraception. Steroids. 2003;68(10-13):809-15.

38. Bassett SG, Little-Ihrig LL, Mason JI, Zeleznik AJ. Expression of messenger ribonucleic acids that encode for 3-hydroxysteroid dehydrogenase and cholesterol side-chain cleavage enzyme throughout the luteal phase of the Macaque menstrual cycle. J Clin Endocrinol Metab. 1991;72:362.
39. Roseff SJ, Bangah ML, Kettel LM, Vale W, Rivier J, Burger HG, et al. Dynamic changes in circulating inhibin levels during the luteal–follicular transition of the human menstrual cycle. J Clin Endocrinol Metab. 1989;69:1033.
40. Jia X-C, Kessel B, Yen SSC, Tucker EM, Hsueh AJW. Serum bioactive follicle-stimulating hormone during the human menstrual cycle and in hyper- and hypogonadotropic states: application of a sensitive granulosa cell aromatase bioassay. J Clin Endocrinol Metab. 1986;62:1243.
41. Schneyer AL, Sluss PM, Whitcomb RW, Hall JE, Crowley Jr WF, Freaman RG. Development of a radioligand receptor assay for measuring follitropin in serum: application to premature ovarian failure. Clin Chem. 1991;37:508.
42. Lehman MN, Coolen LM, Goodman RL. Minireview: kisspeptin/neurokinin B/dynorphin (KNDy) cells of the arcuate nucleus: a central node in the control of gonadotropin-releasing hormone secretion. Endocrinology. 2010;151(8):3479-89.
43. Navarro VM. New insights into the control of pulsatile GnRH release: the role of Kiss1/neurokinin B neurons. Front Endocrinol. 2012;3:48.

Chapter 2

Ovarian Reserve Testing: An Update

Padma Rekha Jirge

■ INTRODUCTION

Ovarian reserve is the quantity of the remaining primordial follicle pool.[1] It declines progressively with age and has practical implications to the fertility potential. It is believed that there is an accelerated decline in the follicle numbers when the critical number reaches 25,000 and fertility remains only for a relatively short period beyond this stage.[2] Poor ovarian reserve is associated with a reduction in the reproductive span. However, the effect of low ovarian reserve on the fertility potential in young women may differ from that seen in older women. The magnitude of decline varies among women of similar age. Hence, assessment of ovarian reserve has become a part of evaluation of infertility in women.

■ OVARIAN RESERVE TESTS

An ideal ovarian reserve test (ORT) should be easy to perform, easily reproducible, noninvasive, accurately measure the quantity and hence quality of the follicular pool, and predict the chances of pregnancy.[3] The ORTs provide an indirect estimation of the ovarian reserve as direct measurement of the size of the primordial follicle pool hitherto has not been possible. They have been developed primarily with an aim to predict the ovarian response in in vitro fertilization (IVF). The commonly considered ORTs are shown in Box 1.[4]

Biological Age

Biological age remains the most important predictor of occurrence of a pregnancy in an individual.[1] It is known that both ovarian reserve and fecundability reduce rapidly after the age of 37 years.[5,6] In those undergoing IVF, most of the embryos are found to be aneuploid by the age of 44 years.[7] This is contrast to that seen in women younger than 35 years of age with poor ovarian response, where most of the embryos are euploid.[8] As there is a wide spectrum of responses encountered in women undergoing IVF from normal to hyper-response, biological age alone cannot be used as a marker of ovarian reserve.

Ovarian Reserve Testing: An Update

BOX 1: Ovarian Reserve Tests.

- *Biological:* Chronological age
- *Biochemical:*
  1. *Static:*
     - FSH
     - Inhibin B
     - Anti-Müllerian hormone (AMH)
     - Estradiol
     - FSH:LH ratio
  2. *Dynamic:*
     - Clomiphene citrate challenge test (CCT)
     - GnRH agonist stimulation test (GAST)
     - Exogenous FSH ovarian reserve test (EFORT)
- *Sonographic paramaters:*
  - Antral follicle count (AFC)
  - Ovarian volume
  - Ovarian vascular flow

Basal Serum Follicle-stimulating Hormone

Basal follicle-stimulating hormone (FSH), measured in the morning on day 2–4 of a cycle, is the most widely used ORT since the 1980s.[9] The measurement of FSH is easy and inexpensive, and a value of 10–12 IU/L is considered as the upper limit of normal range. However, it has diurnal, intra-, and inter-cycle variability.[10] Progressive follicular depletion results in increasing levels of FSH. In women with regular menstrual cycles, FSH can predict poor ovarian response only at very high levels and consequently is helpful to only a small number of women as a screening test for poor ovarian reserve. Considering that decline in ovarian reserve begins several years earlier to any elevation in serum FSH levels, a normal value cannot rule out a poor ovarian response.[11] Hence, in the current clinical scenario, FSH cannot be used alone to predict ovarian reserve.

Serum Estradiol

An elevated serum estradiol (E2) level may mask abnormal FSH levels and the ovarian reserve may be wrongly considered as normal.[12] Hence, addition of serum E2 values on day 2–4 of the cycle with FSH values is considered to reflect ovarian reserve more precisely. Elevated basal E2 in itself (>80 pg/mL) is also considered as a predictor of poor response.[12] However, a meta-analysis concluded that basal E2 does not add to the predictive value of other ORTs; hence, it should not be used in routine clinical practice as an ORT.[11]

Serum Inhibin B

Inhibin B is a glycoprotein produced in the granulosa cells of ovarian follicles. A serum inhibin B level of <45 pg/mL predicts poor response to ovarian stimulation for IVF.[13] It was the first ORT used to predict hyper-response in IVF. However, unreliability of the assays and availability of more robust markers of ovarian reserve, such as anti-Müllerian hormone (AMH), have limited the use of inhibin B as an ORT in recent years.

Serum Anti-Müllerian Hormone

Anti-Müllerian hormone is a dimeric glycoprotein exclusively produced by granulosa cells of preantral and small antral follicles (AFs) in the ovary.[14] It is produced by the granulosa cells of the follicles following their transition from primordial pool to the primary stage and continues till the follicles reach the antral stage with diameters of 2–6 mm. These small AFs reflect the size of the primordial pool. As the size of the follicular pool declines with age, AMH production diminishes and becomes undetectable at menopause.[15] It is a regulator of follicular recruitment and with declining AMH levels, there is an accelerated loss of follicles.[16] The earliest AMH assays were semiautomated; however, the fully automated assays, which are currently used, have reduced the time consumed for performing the assay and made international comparison feasible.

The following paragraph summarizes certain advantages of AMH over other ORTs:[17-22]

- It shows minimal intra- and inter-cycle variability, and hence can be measured on any day of the menstrual cycle.
- It is the earliest marker to show decline in ovarian reserve. Levels below 1.26 ng/mL are considered to indicate poor ovarian response to ovarian stimulation. At levels of 0.5–1.26 ng/mL, AMH indicates perimenopausal transition within 3–5 years. Such women still have a favorable outcome with IVF if the treatment is prioritized.
- It is a very sensitive marker to predict hyper-response in IVF.
- It may be used as a screening test in a general subfertile population to identify those with poor ovarian reserve.
- Serum AMH levels strongly correlate with antral follicle count (AFC) measured by transvaginal ultrasonography (TVS).
- Age-related population nomograms are available for AMH and this provides an opportunity to counsel young women with low AMH regarding prioritizing conception or for oocyte cryopreservation.
- AMH is the only ovarian reserve marker found to be reliable in assessing the residual ovarian reserve in young cancer survivors who have received gonadotoxic therapy previously.
- Whether AMH can predict the occurrence of pregnancy is less clear. However, recent evidence suggests that AMH may be a better predictor of occurrence of pregnancy in young poor responders than age alone.

Dynamic Tests

Three dynamic tests have been used in the past to assess ovarian reserve.[23] They are time consuming, expensive, and are inferior to the more robust markers such as AMH and AFC. Their use in routine clinical practice is no longer recommended.

1. *Clomiphene citrate challenge test* (*CCCT*): This involves estimating basal FSH level on day 3 followed by administration of 100 mg of clomiphene from day 5 to day 9 and estimation of FSH level on day 10. Either an abnormally high basal FSH or an abnormally high value of cumulative FSH (day 3 + day 10) is considered as evidence of poor ovarian reserve.
2. *Exogenous follicle-stimulating hormone ovarian reserve test* (*EFORT*): This involves estimation of basal FSH and E2 on day 3 of the cycle followed by administration of 300 IU FSH on the same day. Serum E2 concentration is rechecked 24 hours later. It was found to be of value in predicting hyper-response, but had a high false-positive rate.
3. *Gonadotropin-releasing hormone agonist stimulation test* (*GAST*): This test involves estimation of day 2 serum E2 followed by administration of gonadotropin-releasing hormone agonist (GnRH-a) (triptorelin 100 µg) subcutaneously. The test is repeated 24 hours later, and an elevation in E2 is considered to indicate good ovarian reserve. It has been used in the past to identify poor responders.

Antral Follicle Count

Antral follicles are all the small follicles in the ovary measuring 2–10 mm in diameter. The AFC is measured in the early follicular phase (day 2–4) using TVS with a 7.5 mHz probe. Two perpendicular measurements are taken of each of the follicles and the mean value is considered as the diameter of the follicle. The follicles in both ovaries are added for the total AFC.[24] An AFC of 8–16 is considered to predict normal ovarian response in IVF, whereas those below <8 are considered to predict poor ovarian response. An AFC of >16 is highly predictive of hyper-response. AFs of 2–6 and 2–9 mm are both considered to reflect AFC. However, the number of AFs of 2–6 mm diameter decline with age, whereas those of 7–9 mm diameter remain constant; hence, the former appears to be a more reliable marker of ovarian reserve. There is limited inter-cycle variability; however, inter-observer variability in young women may be high. Use of three-dimensional (3D) ultrasound does not have any advantage over two-dimensional (2D) ultrasound in the assessment of ovarian reserve.

Antral follicle count has a strong correlation with AMH and has similar sensitivity and specificity to predict both poor and hyper-response. Current evidence does not support its ability to predict occurrence of pregnancy.

Ovarian Volume

Ovarian volume is measured by TVS using the formula for an ellipsoid. Even though increased ovarian volume is an important diagnostic criterion for polycystic ovary syndrome (PCOS), it does not add to the predictive value of AFC while assessing ovarian reserve.[25]

Ovarian Biopsy

Biopsy of ovarian cortex obtained during laparoscopy or laparotomy has shown declining follicular density with age. However, the follicles are not uniformly distributed in the cortex; hence, the biopsy may not represent the true follicular density.[26] In addition, any such invasive procedure has no place in the current clinical scenario in the presence of ovarian reserve markers such as AMH and AFC.

OVARIAN RESERVE TESTING: CURRENT PRACTICE AND UTILITY

Historically, ORTs were developed to provide prognostic information for IVF cycles.[1] There are four important areas where ORTs aid in decision-making:

1. *IVF:* AMH and AFC help in individualizing the protocol and FSH dosing. They provide an opportunity to counsel couples regarding expected poor or hyper-response and their implications.[27] A raised FSH with low AMH or AFC further supports the occurrence of poor response in IVF.
2. *Subfertile women:* In women undergoing expectant management or simple forms of infertility treatment, an abnormally elevated FSH or low AMH and AFC unmask poor ovarian reserve. Such women may be counseled regarding fast-tracking of their treatment to maximize their chances of achieving pregnancy with their own eggs.
3. *General population:* In women who wish to delay conception, particularly in populations where nomograms are available, those with AMH values along the lower centiles may be advised to prioritize pregnancy or to consider oocyte cryopreservation.
4. *Young cancer survivors:* As the survival rates from various malignancies during childhood and in young adults improve, fertility becomes important for many of these young cancer survivors. AMH is shown to be a reliable marker for assessing residual ovarian function in such women.

Even though there is general consensus that ORTs predict the quantity of follicles reliably, there is controversy regarding their ability to predict the quality of oocytes and hence the occurrence of pregnancy. Age is generally considered the best measure of oocyte quality and young women with reduced quantity of oocytes still have a good pregnancy outcome.[14] However, recent evidence has challenged this view and suggests that a low AMH and AFC may also be indicative of poor oocyte quality.[27]

Ovarian reserve test assessment should be postponed if there is history of oral contraceptive pill use. In addition, cigarette smoking and certain ethnicities including Indian ethnicity are associated with lower ovarian reserve.[28] AMH has also allowed exploration of an association between poor ovarian reserve and genetic factors such as *BRCA* mutations or environmental toxins such as bisphenol A and phthalate.[28-30]

CONCLUSION

Ovarian reserve tests play an important role in the evaluation of infertile women. AMH and AFC have the best predictive value for ovarian reserve compared to all other markers. Age is considered to be the most important factor in predicting the occurrence of pregnancy. In the current scenario, a basal FSH and E2 and AMH or AFC provide adequate assessment of ovarian reserve. AMH, in addition, is proven to be a good screening test for general population wishing to delay fertility and also to identify poor responders in the subfertile population to expedite and fast-track the treatment.

KEY MESSAGES
- ORTs form an important part of evaluation of female fertility.
- FSH has limited role in assessing ovarian reserve except when the levels are increased.
- AMH and AFC predict normal, hyper-, or poor response with high sensitivity and specificity.
- AMH may be the earliest marker to identify declining ovarian reserve under certain special circumstances.

REFERENCES

1. Practice Committee of the American Society for Reproductive Medicine. Testing and interpreting measures of ovarian reserve: a committee opinion. Fertil Steril. 2020;114(6):1151-7.
2. Nikolaou D, Templeton A. Early ovarian ageing: a hypothesis. Detection and clinical relevance. Hum Reprod. 2003;18(6):1137-9.
3. de Carvalho BR, Rosa e Silva AC, Rosa e Silva JC, dos Reis RM, Ferriani RA, Silva de Sá MF. Ovarian reserve evaluation: state of the art. J Assist Reprod Genet. 2008;25(7):311-22.
4. Jirge PR. Ovarian reserve tests. J Hum Reprod Sci. 2011;4(3):108-13.
5. Wood JW. Fecundity and natural fertility in humans. Oxf Rev Reprod Biol. 1989;11:61-109.
6. Sharif K, Elgendy M, Lashen H, Afnan M. Age and basal follicle stimulating hormone as predictors of in vitro fertilisation outcome. Br J Obstet Gynaecol. 1998;105:107-12.
7. Franasiak JM, Forman EJ, Hong KH, Werner MD, Upham KM, Treff NR, et al. The nature of aneuploidy with increasing age of the female partner: a review of 15,169 consecutive trophectoderm biopsies evaluated with comprehensive chromosomal screening. Fertil Steril. 2014;101(3):656-63.

8. Bishop LA, Richter KS, Patounakis G, Andriani L, Moon K, Devine K. Diminished ovarian reserve as measured by means of baseline follicle-stimulating hormone and antral follicle count is not associated with pregnancy loss in younger in vitro fertilization patients. Fertil Steril. 2017;108:980-7.
9. Scott RT, Toner JP, Muasher SJ, Oehninger S, Robinson S, Rosenwaks Z. Follicle-stimulating hormone levels on cycle day 3 are predictive of in vitro fertilization outcome. Fertil Steril. 1989;51(4):651-4.
10. Kwee J, Schats R, McDonnell J, Lambalk CB, Schoemaker J. Intercycle variability of ovarian reserve tests: results of a prospective randomized study. Hum Reprod. 2004;19:590-5.
11. Broekmans FJ, Kwee J, Hendriks DJ, Mol BW, Lambalk CB. A systematic review of tests predicting ovarian reserve and IVF outcome. Hum Reprod Update. 2006;12:685-718.
12. Evers JL, Slaats P, Land JA, Dumoulin JC, Dunselman GA. Elevated levels of basal estradiol-17β predict poor response in patients with normal basal levels of follicle-stimulating hormone undergoing in vitro fertilization. Fertil Steril. 1998;69:1010-4.
13. Seifer DB, Lambert-Messerlian G, Hogan JW, Gardiner AC, Blazar AS, Berk CA. Day 3 serum inhibin-B is predictive of assisted reproductive technologies outcome. Fertil Steril. 1997;67(1):110-4.
14. Feyereisen E, Méndez Lozano DH, Taieb J, Hesters L, Frydman R, Fanchin R. Anti-Müllerian hormone: clinical insights into a promising biomarker of ovarian follicular status. Reprod Biomed Online. 2006;12(6):695-703.
15. de Vet A, Laven JS, de Jong FH, Themmen AP, Fauser BC. Anti-Müllerian hormone serum levels: a putative marker for ovarian aging. Fertil Steril. 2002;77:357-62.
16. Weenen C, Laven JS, Von Bergh AR, Cranfield M, Groome NP, Visser JA, et al. Anti-Müllerian hormone expression pattern in the human ovary: potential implications for initial and cyclic follicle recruitment. Mol Hum Reprod. 2004;10:77-83.
17. Hehenkamp WJ, Looman CW, Themmen AP, de Jong FH, te Velde ER, Broekmans FJ. Anti-Müllerian hormone levels in the spontaneous menstrual cycle do not show substantial fluctuation. J Clin Endocrinol Metab. 2006;10:4057-63.
18. Gnoth C, Schuring AN, Friol K, Tigges J, Mallmann P, Godehardt E. Relevance of anti-Mullerian hormone measurement in a routine IVF program. Hum Reprod. 2008;23:1359-65.
19. Fleming R, Seifer DB, Frattarelli JL, Ruman J. Assessing ovarian response: antral follicle count versus anti-Müllerian hormone. Reprod Biomed Online. 2015;31(4):486-96.
20. Nelson SM, Messow MC, Wallace AM, Fleming R, McConnachie A. Nomogram for the decline in serum antimüllerian hormone: a population study of 9,601 infertility patients. Fertil Steril. 2011;95(2):736-41.
21. Martyn F, O'Brien YM, Wingfield M. Review of clinical indicators, including serum anti-Müllerian hormone levels, for identification of women who should consider egg freezing. Int J Gynaecol Obstet. 2017;138(1):37-41.
22. Charpentier AM, Chong AL, Gingras-Hill G, Ahmed S, Cigsar C, Gupta AA, et al. Anti-Müllerian hormone screening to assess ovarian reserve among female survivors of childhood cancer. J Cancer Surviv. 2014;8(4):548-54.

23. Maheshwari A, Fowler P, Bhattacharya S. Assessment of ovarian reserve—should we perform tests of ovarian reserve routinely? Hum Reprod. 2006;21:2729-35.
24. Broekmans FJ, de Ziegler D, Howles CM, Gougeon A, Trew G, Olivennes F. The antral follicle count: practical recommendations for better standardization. Fertil Steril. 2010;94:1044-51.
25. Hendriks DJ, Kwee J, Mol BW, te Velde ER, Broekmans FJ. Ultrasonography as a tool for the prediction of outcome in IVF patients: a comparative meta-analysis of ovarian volume and antral follicle count. Fertil Steril. 2007;87:764-75.
26. Sharara FI, Scott RT. Assessment of ovarian reserve. Is there still a role for ovarian biopsy? First do no harm! Hum Reprod. 2004;19:470-1.
27. Tal R, Seifer DB, Tal R, Granger E, Wantman E, Tal O. AMH highly correlates with cumulative live birth rate in women with diminished ovarian reserve independent of age. J Clin Endocrinol Metab. 2021;106(9):2754-66.
28. Gromski PS, Patil RS, Chougule SM, Bhomkar DA, Jirge PR, Nelson SM. Ethnic discordance in serum anti-Müllerian hormone in European and Indian healthy women and Indian infertile women. Reprod Biomed Online. 2022;45(5):979-86.
29. Turan V, Lambertini M, Lee DY, Wang E, Clatot F, Karlan BY, et al. Association of germline BRCA pathogenic variants with diminished ovarian reserve: a meta-analysis of individual patient-level data. J Clin Oncol. 2021;39(18):2016-24.
30. Park SY, Jeon JH, Jeong K, Chung HW, Lee H, Sung YA, et al. The association of ovarian reserve with exposure to bisphenol A and phthalate in reproductive-aged women. J Korean Med Sci. 2021;36(2):e1.

Chapter 3

Polycystic Ovarian Syndrome

Jwal Banker, Duru Shah

■ INTRODUCTION

Polycystic ovarian syndrome (PCOS), a complex genetic condition, is a highly prevalent heterogeneous syndrome of clinical and/or biochemical androgen excess, ovulatory dysfunction, and polycystic ovarian morphology (PCOM). Stein and Leventhal were pioneers in describing menstrual dysfunction, PCOM, and androgenic features as a part of a condition in 1935. Following that, many other classifications have been formed.[1] The key diagnostic features of PCOS are hyperandrogenemia/hyperandrogenism, oligoanovulation, and PCOM. The three popularly used criteria for defining PCOS have utilized different combinations of these features.[2-4]

From an evolutionary aspect, PCOS evolved as a means of preserving anabolism and reproductive capacity in times of nutritional deprivation. The higher androgen levels of such women would have been advantageous to reproduction as well as survival, but in current times of plenty, this has its disadvantages.[5] The vast miscellany of apparently unrelated gene variations that are associated with PCOS suggests it to be a disorder with contributions from both heritable factors and congenital and acquired factors that affect ovarian steroidogenesis. Studies show that epigenetic changes in fetal life have a role in the developmental origins of PCOS. It has been shown that early prenatal testosterone-treated female rhesus monkeys have reduced hypothalamic steroid negative feedback and hence show luteinizing hormone (LH) hypersecretion. These female monkeys exhibited ovarian hyperandrogenism, oligoanovulation, insulin resistance, and PCOM.[6] Clinical data have yet to verify that excessive testosterone in humans during early development can cause PCOS. Studies do cast a doubt, but do not rule out the role of androgen exposure during early intrauterine life in the occurrence of PCOS.

The PCOS ovary is a topic of great interest due to its varied appearance. Its appearance can be just like a normal ovary or can be a polycystic one with the typical morphology and characteristics. In most cases, folliculogenesis is disturbed due to various endocrine and paracrine factors. In spite of the

Polycystic Ovarian Syndrome

advances in diagnostic science, the exact etiology and mechanism are still an enigma, though various theories are postulated.

■ FOLLICULOGENESIS IN NORMAL OVARIES

It is well established that normal ovarian folliculogenesis is required for regular menstruation, ovulation, and fertility. During ovarian follicular development, only selected follicles are recruited and start growing from a cohort of primordial follicles. One growing follicle attains dominance and finally ovulates.

All steps starting with the recruitment of a dominant follicle from the primordial follicles, its growth, and ultimate ovulation require complex interactions between the metabolic and the reproductive functions. Intraovarian paracrine signals coordinate and are responsible for granulosa cell proliferation, theca cell differentiation, and even oocyte maturation. The follicles in ovaries are broadly divided into two stages: *Preantral follicles* (primordial, primary, secondary, tertiary) and *antral follicles* (graafian, small, medium, large, preovulatory). Early follicle development to an initial antral stage is relatively independent of gonadotropins and relies mostly on intrinsic mesenchymal–epithelial cell interactions, intraovarian paracrine signals, and oocyte-secreted factors. Beyond this stage, antral follicle development and differentiation depend upon circulating gonadotropins in combination with these locally derived regulators **(Fig. 1)**.[7]

Initially, the primordial follicle consists of an oocyte at the diplotene stage of prophase one surrounded by squamous granulosa cells. As the primordial follicle grows, its oocyte synthesizes ribonucleic acid (RNA), and its squamous granulosa cells become a single layer of cuboidal and mixed squamous granulosa cells (the intermediate follicle) or a single layer of cuboidal granulosa cells entirely (the primary follicle).[8] A secondary follicle is formed with the progressive multiplication of the granulosa cell into multiple layers. Theca cells are recruited from surrounding stromal stem cells and are organized into distinct theca cell layers around the follicle, establishing mesenchymal–epithelial cell interactions that promote development of the follicle and its oocyte. To promote the subsequent development of the follicle

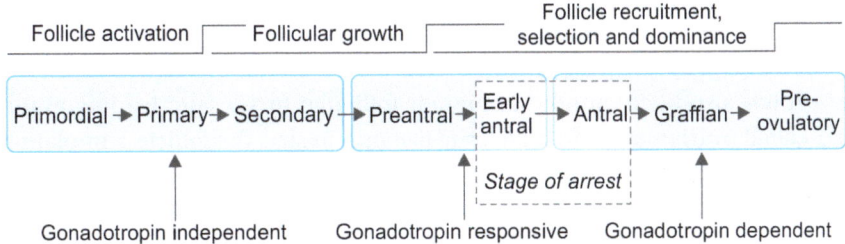

Fig. 1: Different stages of follicular growth and its interaction with gonadotropins.

and its oocyte, theca cells are recruited from the surrounding stromal cells and these cells organize themselves around the follicle to create a mesenchymal–epithelial cell relationship for signaling.

In the last stage of recruitment, an antral follicle is formed that contains extracellular fluid and mural and cumulus cell layers, which are formed from the granulosa cells. This antral follicle becomes primarily responsive to gonadotropins and is 2–5 mm in size. Each month, one such follicle normally becomes dominant and eventually ovulates.[9] It is noteworthy that in women of reproductive age, more than a 100 primordial follicles initiate growth, out of which about 10–20 selected antral follicles remain at the beginning of the normal cycle, but ultimately only one normally continues to grow and ovulate.

The process of recruitment of follicles, growth, and the selection of the dominant follicle is disturbed in women with PCOS. Ovarian hyperandrogenism, hyperinsulinemia from insulin resistance, and altered intrafollicular paracrine signaling contribute to the accumulation of small antral follicles within the periphery of the ovary, giving it a polycystic morphology. Studies show that increased recruitment from primordial follicles to growing follicles is a characteristic factor in PCOS, which causes the typical PCOM.

INCREASED FOLLICULAR RECRUITMENT AND LATER FOLLICULAR ARREST

A distinctive feature of the polycystic ovary (PCO) is an increase in follicle number as the population of growing preantral and antral follicles exceeds by two- to threefold that of normal ovaries. In an interesting study, Webber et al. studied the histology of follicles in women with and without PCOS. They commented that the increased density of follicles in adult PCO suggests that such ovaries were characterized by a greater initial pool of follicles. Analysis of the proportions of primordial and primary follicles indicated that, irrespective of ovulation status, there might be an increased recruitment from the primordial resting follicle pool in PCO. The proportion of atretic follicles in ovulatory or anovulatory PCO did not differ from that in normal ovaries.[10] An alternative explanation can also be that the growth of preantral follicles occurs more slowly in PCOS, leading to an accumulation of growing follicles **(Fig. 2)**.

It has also been found that there is follicular arrest later leading to the so-called ovarian cysts. In follicles of 6–8 mm in size, the follicle-stimulating hormone (FSH)-stimulated granulosa cells begin to express cytochrome P450 aromatase, which help androgens produced by LH-stimulated theca cells to undergo aromatization to estrogens. The theca cells contain $P450_{c17}$, a rate-limiting step in androgen synthesis, which regulates whether androgens

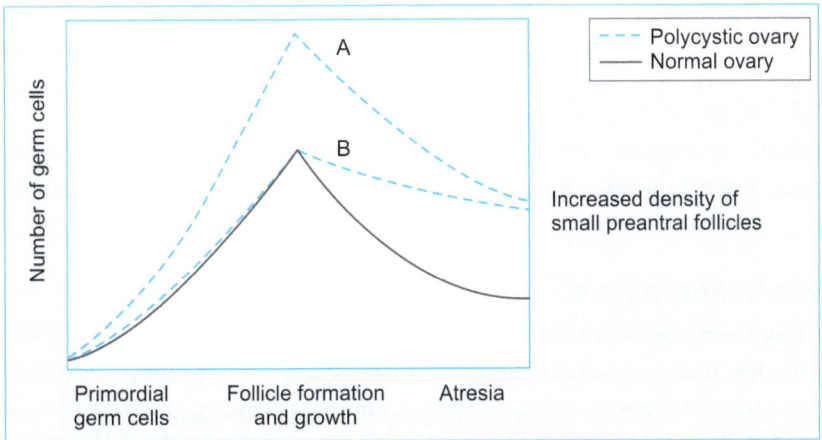

A: ?Higher initial population of primodial follicles, ?More cell divisions and growth
B: ?Slower rate of atresia

Fig. 2: Possible changes leading to the typical polycystic ovarian morphology.
Source: Adapted from Webber LJ, et al. (2003).[10]

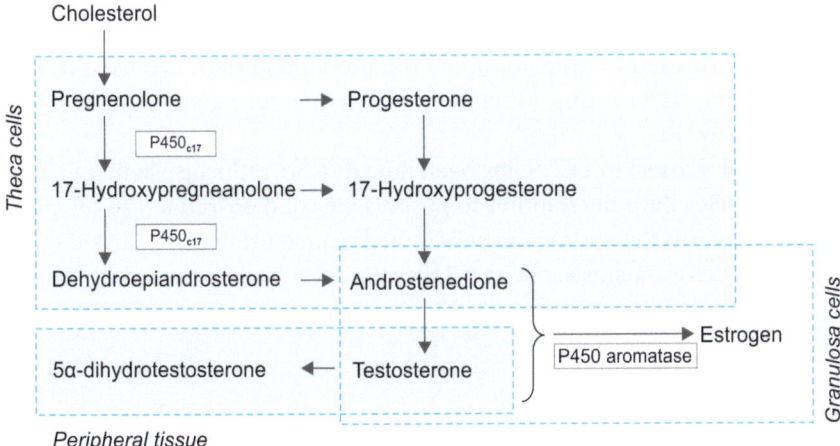

Fig. 3: Simplified illustration demonstrating the role of $P450_{c17}$ and P450 aromatase in steroid metabolism.

or progestins are produced in the steroid pathway **(Fig. 3)**. Progesterone can be hydroxylated by $P450_{c17}$ to form 17α-hydroxyprogesterone that is then converted to androstenedione. Also, dehydroepiandrosterone (DHEA) is converted to testosterone by the action of 17β-hydroxysteroid dehydrogenase. These potent androgens, testosterone and androstenedione, are taken up by granulosa cells, where the P450 aromatase, under the control of FSH, converts them into estrogen, thus raising the estrogen levels. The peripheral tissues contain 5α-reductase, which converts testosterone to a more potent form known as 5α-dihydrotestosterone. This potent androgen is assumed to cause symptoms of hyperandrogenism in PCOS women. Follicular arrest in PCOS occurs at this stage when granulosa cells normally begin to express aromatase, causing secretion of excessive estrogens and hampering the feedback mechanisms. This might be responsible for the menstrual irregularity, anovulatory subfertility, and the accumulation of small antral follicles within the periphery of the ovarian cortex, giving it a polycystic morphology.[11-13]

Role of Androgens

It has been thought that androgens promote early follicular growth in primates. Weil et al. supplemented testosterone in adult rhesus monkeys and found that there was an increase in the number of primary, growing preantral and small antral follicles. There was also an increase in the proliferation of granulosa cells within them by acting through its own receptors.[14] This potential of androgens to initiate the growth of follicles is also supported by the observations that the androstenedione levels in the follicular fluid are increased in ovulatory women with PCO. It is also found that androstenedione secretion by their cultured theca cells is increased.[15] Another interesting study demonstrated multifollicular ovarian development in sheep who were exposed to testosterone in the prenatal period.[16] Hence, there is quite some evidence supporting the role of hyperandrogenism in increased follicular growth.

Follicular arrest in PCOS has been linked to 5α-reductase activity. Small PCOS follicles have been found to possess elevated 5α-reductase function, which increases the androgen levels to high concentrations, obstructing the granulosa cell aromatase activity.[17] This ultimately leads to cyst-like follicular formation and the appearance of PCOM.

Role of Insulin

Insulin has been linked to functions such as glucose uptake, protein synthesis, and steroidogenesis. Insulin receptors have been identified on theca cells, granulosa cells, oocytes, and even the surrounding stroma. This insulin can act either alone or as a co-stimulant and stimulate theca cell androgen production and amplify LH-stimulated granulosa cell estrogen and progesterone production.[18]

There is an intrinsic dysfunction in insulin sensitivity in women with PCOS. The hyperinsulinemia has been found to promote androgen production in the ovaries by stimulating theca cell 17α-hydroxylase activity, boosting insulin-like growth factor-1 (IGF-1)-stimulated androgen production and increasing free testosterone by reducing hepatic sex binding globulin.[19] Hyperinsulinemia is also associated and responsible for the premature luteinization seen in PCO. When granulosa cells from small follicles in women with PCOS were cultured with LH, it was found that there was hypersecretion of progesterone and overexpression of LH receptors, which ultimately causes a shift in steroidogenesis from estrogen to progesterone production.[20,21] Hence, insulin, either directly or indirectly via androgens, promotes follicular growth.

Role of Anti-Müllerian Hormone

Anti-Müllerian hormone (AMH) belongs to the transforming growth factor beta (TGF-β) superfamily. This AMH is normally produced by the granulosa cells of large preantral and early antral follicles. It is evident that PCOS ovaries comprise a higher number of preantral and small antral follicles, during which phase the AMH production is usually highest. It has been found that serum AMH levels, independent of antral follicle number, are elevated in normoandrogenic women with PCO and are further increased in hyperandrogenic women with PCO. In addition, the concentration of AMH in follicular fluid from women with anovulatory PCOS was found to be much greater compared with ovulatory women.[22]

It is thought that AMH regulation might have a role in PCOS. Studies on rodents have also found that AMH inhibits primordial follicle growth and further follicular maturation. The proposed mechanism of this reciprocal inhibition is as mentioned in **Figure 4**. Theories also suggest that the AMH produced by these growing follicles might inhibit the further growth of even adjacent primordial follicles. In an interesting study, it was shown that granulosa cells of PCO have increased AMH micro-RNA (mRNA) expression, which can lead to its overproduction.[23] Hence, overproduction of AMH by the granulosa cells of ovarian follicles in PCOS appears to antagonize FSH action in small PCOS follicles, and such follicles are estrogen depleted even if there is sufficient FSH available. It is quite possible that the follicular cysts seen in PCOM may be due to this factor and that these follicles fail to mature.[24-28]

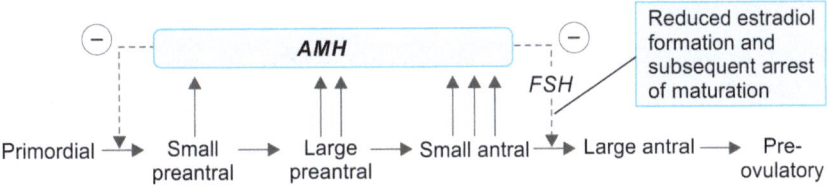

The inhibitory actions of AMH are shown on the FSH-independent initial recruitment of primary follicles from the primordial follicle pool and on the FSH-dependent follicular maturation and selection of the dominant follicle by decreasing follicular sensitivity to FSH. AMH inhibits FSH-induced aromatase expression in granulosa cells, reducing the conversion of testosterone to estradiol, which in turn inhibits AMH.

Fig. 4: Role of anti-Müllerian hormone (AMH) in the pathophysiology of polycystic ovary (PCO). (FSH: follicle-stimulating hormone)

■ IMAGING WITH ULTRASOUND

The original Rotterdam criteria introduced the concept of ovaries with PCOM. The parameters in establishing the criteria were based on a single report comparing it with controls. The initial criteria in defining PCOM were 12 or more follicles measuring 2-9 mm throughout the entire ovary or an ovarian volume ≥10 cubic cm.[4] This stood true for that era where imaging modality was primitive compared to recent time. Nowadays, there was a need for modification due to several reasons as mentioned in **Box 1**.

The latest ESHRE-Monash University guidelines analyzed the available literature for this purpose. Due to heterogeneity in threshold/cutoff values of different parameters, analysis was done by creating forest plots from available data. Eleven studies, analyzing data of more than 2,500 women, suggested a cut-off value of >19 follicle number per ovary (FNPO) with an optimal sensitivity. For ovarian volume, data from more than 2,000 participants were assessed, but showed different outcomes suggesting sensitivity for both 5-8 cubic cm as well as 9-10 cubic cm. One is also advised to keep in mind that PCOM criteria of adults are likely to be inaccurate for ultrasound diagnosis of PCOS in adolescence due to substantive overlap between follicle numbers per ovary in normal adolescents and those with other features of PCOS.[29]

The guidelines have laid down certain recommendations which are as mentioned:
- Using transvaginal ultrasound transducers with a frequency bandwidth that includes 8 MHz, the threshold for PCOM should be on either ovary, an FNPO of ≥20, and/or an ovarian volume ≥10 cubic cm, making sure that no corpus luteum, cysts, or dominant follicles are present.
- If using an older technology or transabdominal scan, this threshold could be just an ovarian volume of ≥10 cubic cm on either ovary.
- Transvaginal approach is much more sensitive and should be preferred in a patient who is sexually active and is acceptable to her.
- Ultrasound should not be used in diagnosing PCOS in those having <8 years after menarche due to high multifollicular ovaries at that stage.

BOX 1: Factors mandating regular revision of the polycystic ovarian morphology (PCOM) criteria.

- Advances in ultrasound technologies
- Better resolution in imaging
- Variable operator skill
- Impact of different approach of transducer (transvaginal vs. abdominal)
- Unclear cut-off between normal ovaries and PCOM
- Inadequate initial evidence
- Lack of standard reporting method
- Age and body habits

- Protocol for reporting must be accurate and clear and should include a minimum of these so that there is uniformity in literature:
  - Last menstrual period
  - Transducer bandwidth frequency
  - Approach used
  - Total FNPO measuring 2–9 mm
  - Three-dimensional (3D) and volume of each ovary
  - Other ovarian and uterine pathologies, cysts, endometrial thickness, dominant follicles >10 mm.

CONCLUSION

The ovary in women with PCOS can be in a variety of presentations. In patients with irregular menstrual cycles and documented hyperandrogenism/features of hyperandrogenemia, an ovarian ultrasound is not necessary for the diagnosis of PCOS; however, ultrasound will identify the complete PCOS phenotype. The overall hormonal imbalance caused due to androgens, insulin, AMH, and other active hormones such as inhibin, along with alterations in cell signaling at a deeper level cause problem in the folliculogenesis. There is accelerated growth of the follicles, which ultimately luteinize earlier at the antral stage giving rise to the cystic appearance of the ovaries. Due to lack in uniformity of available literature and difficulty in diagnosing the cause of this complex condition, this syndrome is still an enigma. Regular and systematic reporting will aid updating or developing guidelines.

KEY MESSAGES

- There are multiple reproductive and metabolic features that define PCOS as a disorder.
- PCOS is characterized by anovulation with clinical (hirsutism/acne) and/or biochemical evidence of androgen excess.
- 6-fold increase in density of pre-antral follicles compared to normal ovary (Webber et al. 2003).
- Large cohort of small follicles are arrested in development but capable of responding to exogenous FSH.
- The origin of PCOS starts from intrauterine life and extends throughout life.
- Hyperandrogenemia and hyperinsulinemia are the main pathology in PCOS.
- The exact etiology is not known but various genetic and environmental factors are involved in its pathogenesis.
- *Two underlying hormonal factors:* Insulin resistance and hyperandrogenemia though it is still controversial as to which is a primary defect.
- Pre-pubertal and pubertal hypothalamic exposure to excess androgens results in impaired inhibition of GnRH pulse frequency by increased nocturnal E2 and P4. This persistent rapid frequency of GnRH pulse secretion results in increased LH and decreased FSH synthesis and secretion with increased secretion of androgens and decreased follicular maturation.

Contd...

Contd...

- Androgens influence insulin sensitivity, dyslipidemia, visceral adiposity and adipocyte function in PCOS.
- *AMH inhibits initial follicle recruitment:* Regulates transition of primordial to primary follicle and FSH-dependent growth and selection of pre-antral and small antral follicles and also down regulates the aromatizing capacity of GC.
- Serum AMH correlates with severity of PCOS and precisely with the severity of hyperandrogenism, oligo-anovulation/amenorrhea and polycystic morphology.
- No single test is diagnostic PCOS should be diagnosis of exclusion.
- The transvaginal ultrasound approach is preferred in the diagnosis of PCOS, if sexually active and if acceptable to the individual being assessed.
- If using lower resolution USG transducers (frequency <8 MHz), the threshold for PCOM should be FNPO of ≥12 and/or ovarian volume of ≥10 mL.
- Using endovaginal USG transducers with frequency bandwidth >8 MHz, the threshold for PCOM should be FNPO of ≥20 and/or an ovarian volume ≥10 mL on either ovary, ensuring no corpora lutea, cysts or dominant follicles are present.

■ REFERENCES

1. Stein IF, Leventhal ML. Amenorrhea associated with bilateral polycystic ovaries. Am J Obstet Gynecol. 1935;29:181-91.
2. Azziz R, Carmina E, Dewailly D, Diamanti-Kandarakis E, Escobar-Morreale HF, Futterweit W, et al. Positions statement: criteria for defining polycystic ovary syndrome as a predominantly hyperandrogenic syndrome: an Androgen Excess Society Guideline. J Clin Endocrinol Metab. 2006;91:4237-45.
3. Zawadzki JK, Dunaif A. Diagnostic criteria for polycystic ovary syndrome: towards a rational approach. Boston: Blackwell Scientific; 1992. pp. 377-84.
4. Rotterdam ESHRE/ASRM-Sponsored PCOS Consensus Workshop Group. Revised 2003 consensus on diagnostic criteria and long-term health risks related to polycystic ovary syndrome. Fertil Steril. 2004;81:19-25.
5. Corbett S, Morin-Papunen L. The polycystic ovary syndrome and recent human evolution. Mol Cell Endocrinol. 2013;373:39-50.
6. Abbott DH, Barnett DK, Levine JE, Padmanabhan V, Dumesic DA, Jacoris S, et al. Endocrine antecedents of polycystic ovary syndrome (PCOS) in fetal and infant prenatally androgenized female rhesus monkeys. Biol Reprod. 2008;79:154-63.
7. Erickson GF. (2009). Follicle growth and development. The Global Library of Women's Medicine. Available from https://www.glowm.com/section-view/heading/Follicle%20Growth%20and%20Development/item/288# [Last accessed November, 2022].
8. Trounson A, Gosden R, Eichenlaub-Ritter U. Biology and Pathology of the Oocyte: Role in Fertility, Medicine and Nuclear Reprograming, 2nd edition. Cambridge: Cambridge University Press; 2012. pp. 1-454.
9. Adashi EY, Rock JA, Rosenwaks Z. Reproductive Endocrinology, Surgery, and Technology. Philadelphia: Lippincott Williams & Wilkins; 1996. p. 54.
10. Webber LJ, Stubbs S, Stark J, Trew GH, Margara R, Hardy K, et al. Formation and early development of follicles in the polycystic ovary. Lancet. 2003;362:1017-21.
11. Hull MG. Epidemiology of infertility and polycystic ovarian disease: endocrinological and demographic studies. Gynecol Endocrinol. 1987;1:235-45.
12. Gougeon A. Regulation of ovarian follicular development in primates: facts and hypotheses. Endocr Rev. 1996;17:121-55.

13. Ashraf S, Nabi M, Rasool Su A, Rashid F, Amin S. Hyperandrogenism in polycystic ovarian syndrome and role of *CYP* gene variants: a review. Egyptian J Med Hum Genet. 2019;20:25.
14. Weil SJ, Vendola K, Zhou J, Adesanya OO, Wang J, Okafor J, et al. Androgen receptor gene expression in the primate ovary: cellular localization, regulation, and functional correlations. J Clin Endocrinol Metab. 1998;83:2479-85.
15. Gilling-Smith C, Willis DS, Beard RW, Franks S. Hypersecretion of androstenedione by isolated thecal cells from polycystic ovaries. J Clin Endocrinol Metab. 1994;79:1158-65.
16. West C, Foster DL, Evans NP, Robinson J, Padmanabhan V. Intra-follicular activin availability is altered in prenatally-androgenized lambs. Mol Cell Endocrinol. 2001;185:51-9.
17. Jakimiuk AJ, Weitsman SR, Magoffin DA. 5α-reductase activity in women with polycystic ovary syndrome. J Clin Endocrinol Metab. 1999;84:2414-8.
18. Balen AH, Conway G, Homburg R, Kegro R. Polycystic ovary syndrome: a Guide to clinical management. London: CRC Press; 2005.
19. Bergh C, Carlsson B, Olsson JH, Selleskog U, Hillensjö T. Regulation of androgen production in cultured human thecal cells by insulin-like growth factor I and insulin. Fertil Steril. 1993;59:323-31.
20. Franks S, Mason H, Willis D. Follicular dynamics in the polycystic ovary syndrome. Mol Cell Endocrinol. 2000;163:49-52.
21. Jakimiuk AJ, Weitsman SR, Navab A, Magoffin DA. Luteinizing hormone receptor, steroidogenesis acute regulatory protein, and steroidogenic enzyme messenger ribonucleic acids are overexpressed in thecal and granulosa cells from polycystic ovaries. J Clin Endocrinol Metab. 2001;86:1318-23.
22. Eldar-Geva T, Margalioth EJ, Gal M, Ben-Chetrit A, Algur N, Zylber-Haran E, et al. Serum anti-Müllerian hormone levels during controlled ovarian hyperstimulation in women with polycystic ovaries with and without hyperandrogenism. Hum Reprod. 2005;20:1814-9.
23. Taieb J, Grynberg M, Pierre A, Arouche N, Massart P, Belville C, Hesters L, Frydman R, Catteau-Jonard S, Fanchin R, Picard JY. FSH and its second messenger cAMP stimulate the transcription of human anti-Müllerian hormone in cultured granulosa cells. Molecular Endocrinology. 2011;25(4):645-55.
24. Mason HD, Willis DS, Beard RW, Winston RM, Margara R, Franks S. Estradiol production by granulosa cells of normal and polycystic ovaries: relationship to menstrual cycle history and concentrations of gonadotropins and sex steroids in follicular fluid. J Clin Endocrinol Metab. 1994;79:1355-60.
25. Erickson GF, Magoffin DA, Garzo VG, Cheung AP, Chang RJ. Granulosa cells of polycystic ovaries: are they normal or abnormal? Hum Reprod. 1992;7:293-9.
26. Pellatt L, Hanna L, Brincat M, Galea R, Brain H, Whitehead S, et al. Granulosa cell production of anti-Müllerian hormone is increased in polycystic ovaries. J Clin Endocrinol Metab. 2007;92:240-5.
27. Garg D, Tal R. The role of AMH in the pathophysiology of polycystic ovarian syndrome. Reprod Biomed Online. 2016;33:15-28.
28. Durlinger ALL, Gruijters MJG, Kramer P, Karels B, Ingraham HA, Nachtigal MW, et al. Anti-Müllerian hormone inhibits initiation of primordial follicle growth in the mouse ovary. Endocrinology. 2002;143:1076-84.
29. Teede HJ, Misso ML, Costello MF, Dokras A, Laven J, Moran L, et al. Recommendations from the international evidence-based guideline for the assessment and management of polycystic ovary syndrome. Hum Reprod. 2018;33:1602-18.

Chapter 4

Ovulation Induction in Non-assisted Reproductive Technology Cycles

Chaitanya Shembekar

■ INTRODUCTION

Infertility treatment is all about ovulation induction. Ovulation induction is of utmost importance in anovulatory cycles. Anovulation can result due to the following:
- Hypogonadotropic hypogonadism—follicle-stimulating hormone (FSH) is low, anti-Müllerian hormone (AMH) is low or normal.
- Hypergonadotropic hypogonadism—FSH is high, AMH is low.
- Normogonadotropic anovulation—normal FSH, high AMH
- Hyperprolactinemia—high prolactin and thyroid-stimulating hormone (TSH).

Apart from the above-mentioned causes, ovarian stimulation is done in ovulatory patients as well. This is routinely done in the treatment of other causes of infertility such as unexplained infertility and male factor infertility.

In short, ovulation induction is for anovulatory cycles and ovarian stimulation is for already ovulating cycles.

Using proper drugs after proper evaluation and investigations at its proper timing is important. The choice of treatment depends on age, BMI, presence of other infertility factors, risk tolerance and available resourses. Lifestyle modification followed by oral ovulogens is always the first line of treatment. If there is either resistance or failure to this therapy, second line treatment includes gonadotropins or LOD in women with PCOS. ART is the third and final line of treatment.

Scheme for OI is demonstrated in **Figure 1**.

▌MONO-OVULATION AND CONTROLLED OVARIAN HYPERSTIMULATION

In anovulation, the aim is to promote the development of a single pre-ovulatory follicle. Mono-ovulation is the aim in anovulatory patients but in other causes of infertility, controlled ovarian stimulation with the formation of multiple follicles and ultimately oocytes is the aim.

Response to ovarian stimulation depends on age, AMH, and antral follicular count (AFC). While AMH and AFC are the most reliable factors

Ovulation Induction in Non-assisted Reproductive Technology Cycles

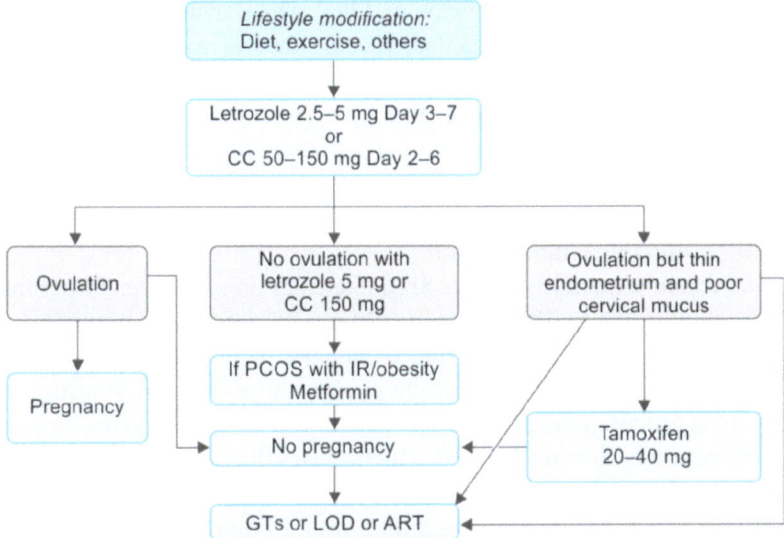

Fig. 1: Algorithm for OI in non-ART cycles.

to decide the dose and type of ovulation induction agent, age and FSH are relatively less reliable as far as the prediction of response is concerned.

Antral follicular count is the sum of antral follicles (2-10 mm) in both ovaries, at a transvaginal ultrasonography during the early follicular phase. A low AFC (range 3-10 total antral follicles) has been associated with poor response to ovarian stimulation and has a lesser chance to achieve pregnancy.[1,2] On the other hand, a high AFC of >20 is associated with a higher chance of developing ovarian hyperstimulation syndrome (OHSS).

- Choice of ovulation induction agent depends upon treatment plan.
- Oral ovulogens are advised in timed intercourse. Oral ovulogens in combination with gonadotropins are given in intrauterine insemination (IUI).
- Injectable gonadotropins are usually advised in cases of IUI.

Ovulation Induction Agents

Oral Ovulogens

Three major molecules in oral ovulogens are: (1) clomiphene citrate (CC); (2) letrozole; and (3) tamoxifen. Metformin is also an oral ovulogen, which works well in combination.

1. *CC:* It is an age-old drug, available since 1960. It is a racemic mixture of Zu 38% cis and En 62% trans-clomiphene. It is antiestrogenic being weak estrogenic in some. It is a selective estrogen receptor modulator (SERM), which when given for 5 days is detected in serum for 30 days. CC is used for various indications such as unexplained infertility, polycystic ovary

(PCO), and luteal phase deficiency (LPD). The starting dose is 50 mg OD for 5 days and the maximum dose is 250. However, most clinicians prefer to start with 100 mg/day. While 75% ovulate with CC, only 40% conceive. This is called CC failure. 25% of the patients do not ovulate and this is called CC resistance. Side effects of CC include mood swings, hot flashes, abdominal and breast discomfort, nausea, vomiting, visual symptoms, headache, OHSS, multiple pregnancy, cyst formation, hostile cervical mucus, and thin endometrium.

2. *Tamoxifen:* It is a nonsteroidal SERM, used in breast cancer. Structurally, it is similar to CC. The dose is 10–20 mg BD for 5 days, ovulation rate is 50–90%, and pregnancy rate is 30–50%. It is found to be good in CC-resistant cases because of the positive effect on endometrium and cervical mucus. Side effects are headache and mild ovarian enlargement.

3. *Letrozole:* It is an oral ovulogen, which causes the conversion of androgen to estrogen under the effect of cytochrome P-dependent enzyme aromatase. It is a competitive inhibitor of aromatase enzyme. It lowers estradiol (E2) levels. It acts in 48–72 hours. Half-life is 48 hours. The conventional dose is 2.5 mg BD for 5 days starting from day 2 of menses. Letrozole is the drug of choice in PCO and is also used in other indications such as endometriosis, unexplained infertility, and male factor infertility. There are many advantages of letrozole over CC. It induces monoovulation, endometrial thickness is better than CC, half-life is less, and so are the chances of OHSS.

ROLE OF GONADOTROPINS IN THE TREATMENT OF INFERTILITY AND INTRAUTERINE INSEMINATION

The rationale for use of gonadotropins in controlled ovarian stimulation is to increase the availability of oocytes and increase steroid production, thus increasing the chance of implantation. If the time period for which FSH remains above the threshold value is extended by administering exogenous FSH in the mid-follicular phase, it results in multifollicular development.[3]

Indications for the Use of Gonadotropins
- CC/letrozole resistance
- CC/letrozole failure
- Persistent hypersecretion of luteinizing hormone (LH)
- IUI and assisted reproductive technology (ART) cycles.

Disadvantages of Gonadotropins
- Cost increases
- Injectable preparations
- Close monitoring is required
- More chances of OHSS.

Gonadotropin preparations that are available are as follows:
- *Urinary* human menopausal gonadotropin (hMG)
- hMG HP (highly purified)
- Urinary FSH
- Recombinant FSH.

OVULATION INDUCTION PROTOCOLS USING GONADOTROPINS

Combination Protocols

Clomiphene Citrate/Tamoxifen + Gonadotropin Protocol (Fig. 2)

Clomiphene citrate 100 mg or tamoxifen 20 mg from day 2 to 6 of menstrual cycle + hMG or FSH 75 IU from day 7 till human chorionic gonadotropin (hCG)

We can also use gonadotropins in the following protocols along with CC and tamoxifen which are given from day 2 to 6.

Gonadotropins can be used as follows:
- On day 3, 5, 7, 9, and 11
- Single-dose hMG/FSH 150 IU on day 9
- hMG/FSH 37.5–75 IU from day 2 onward and dose titrated depending on the response
- hMG/FSH 75 IU given from day 5 onward daily.

Disadvantages: Clomiphene citrate/tamoxifen + gonadotropin
- 20% patients have premature LH surge with a high incidence of premature oocyte maturation.
- Higher incidence of OHSS.
- Higher incidence of multiple pregnancies.

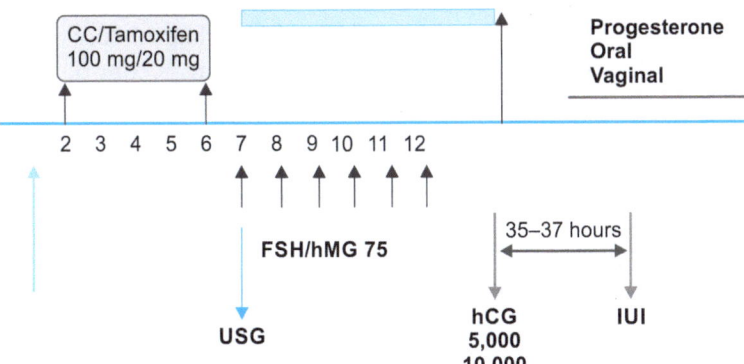

Fig. 2: Clomiphene citrate (CC) + human menopausal gonadotropin (hMG)/follicle-stimulating hormone (FSH). (hCG: human chorionic gonadotropin; IUI: intrauterine insemination; USG: ultrasonography)

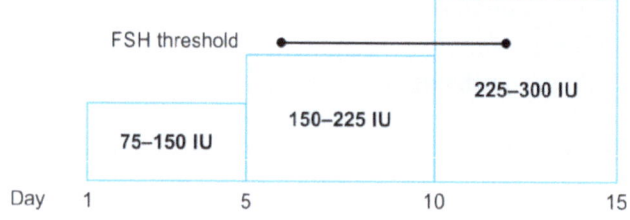

Fig. 3: Conventional step-up protocol. (FSH: follicle-stimulating hormone)

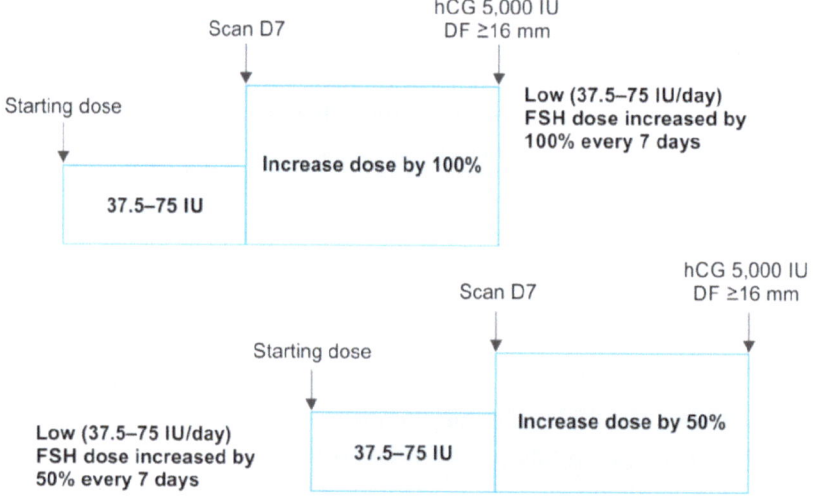

Fig. 4: Low-dose protocol. (DF: dominant follicle; FSH: follicle-stimulating hormone; hCG: human chorionic gonadotropin)

hMG/FSH/Recombinant FSH

Conventional step-up protocol (Fig. 3): Suprophysiological doses of FSH in this protocol provoke initial development of a large cohort, stimulate additional follicles, and even rescue those follicles destined for atresia.

Following are the results with conventional protocol:
- *Ovulation rate:* 70%
- *Severe OHSS:* 7–14%
- *Cumulative pregnancy rate:* 21–75%
- *Multiple pregnancy rate:* 36%.

Low-dose protocol (Fig. 4): Gonadotropins are started in a dose of 37.5–75 IU from day 2 and the first increment in the dose is done on day 7 of stimulation by either 50 or 100% depending on the follicular growth. With this protocol, one can achieve monofolliculogenesis and reduce the risk of OHSS and multiple pregnancies.

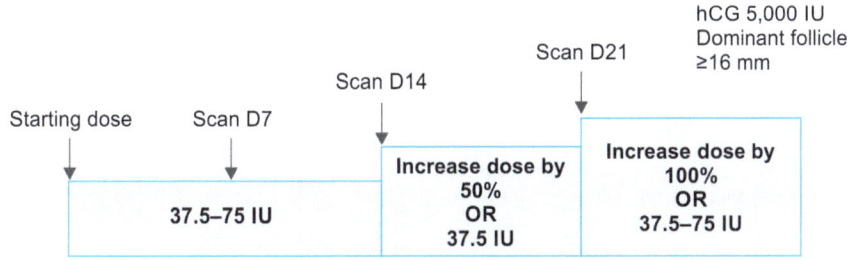

Fig. 5: Chronic low-dose protocol. (hCG: human chorionic gonadotropin; OHSS: ovarian hyperstimulation syndrome)

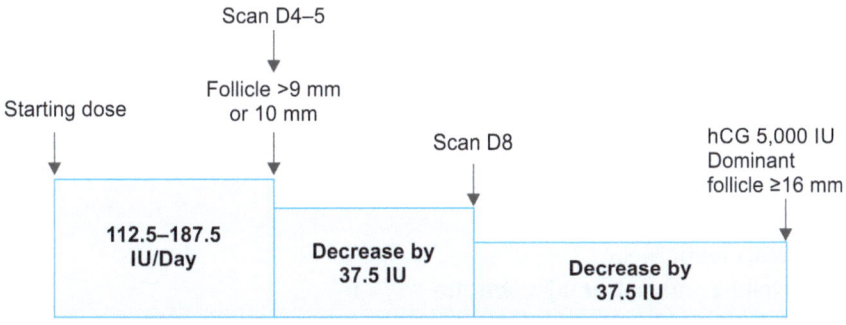

Fig. 6: Step-down protocol. (hCG: human chorionic gonadotropin)

Chronic low-dose protocol (Fig. 5):
- Low (37.5–75 IU/day) FSH dose is increased by 50% or 37.5 IU after 14 days, if no ovarian response.
- Any further FSH increment thereafter is made by 37.5–75 IU at weekly intervals to a maximum of 225 IU/day.
- Once the dominant follicle emerges, the dose of FSH is maintained the same until the follicle reaches 18–20 mm.

Step-down protocol (Fig. 6): Loading FSH dose (112.5–187.5 IU/day) is decreased by 37.5 IU every 3–5 days till dominant follicle emerges. Thereafter, the FSH dose is maintained the same till criteria for administration of hCG are reached.

Sequential protocol (Fig. 7): The basic principle for using the sequential protocol is as follows:
- FSH dependence of the leading follicle decreases as follicle grows.
- Reduction in FSH threshold contributes to the escape of the leading follicle from atresia when FSH concentrations start to decrease due to negative feedback of rising E2.

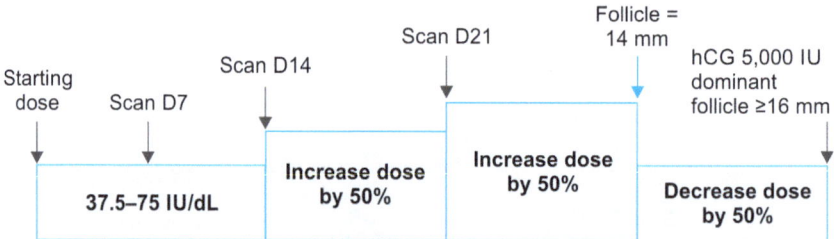

Fig. 7: Sequential protocol. (FSH: follicle-stimulating hormone; hCG: human chorionic gonadotropin; OHSS: ovarian hyperstimulation syndrome)

Stimulation is started with low (37.5–75 IU/day) FSH dose, which is increased by 50% or 37.5 IU after 14 days if no ovarian response is obtained. Thereafter, any further FSH increment is made by 37.5–75 IU at weekly intervals to a maximum of 225 IU/day. Once the dominant follicle emerges and reaches a diameter of 14 mm, the dose is reduced by 50%.

Common side effects of gonadotropins are:
- Multiple pregnancy (25%)
- Breast tenderness
- Swelling and rash at injection site
- Abdominal bloating
- Depression and mood swings
- Mild-to-severe OHSS
- Miscarriage and premature deliveries.

■ CONTRAINDICATIONS TO GONADOTROPIN THERAPY
- Tumors of ovary, breast, pituitary, or hypothalamus
- Pregnancy or lactation
- Undiagnosed vaginal bleeding
- Primary ovarian failure
- Ovarian cyst
- Malformation of sexual organs/fibroid uterus incompatible to pregnancy.

Disadvantages of Controlled Ovarian Hyperstimulation
- It is time consuming and stressful to the couple.
- It imposes a heavy financial burden.
- May cause OHSS, which may be life threatening
- Detrimental effects on embryo implantation due to altered estrogen–progesterone balance can occur.
- Higher incidence of multiple pregnancy with complications such as preterm delivery is encountered

- Eightfold higher incidence of abortions even in singleton pregnancies has been observed.
- Women undergoing ovulation induction agents and especially those women who have landed up in OHSS are at increasing risk of thromboembolism.

Abnormal response to controlled ovarian stimulation includes:
- Premature luteinization
- Endogenous surge
- Poor response
- Hyperstimulation.

Induction of Follicular Maturation and Ovulation

Drugs used for the induction of follicular maturation and ovulation are given at a follicular diameter of 16–18 mm. They are as follows:
- hCG 5,000–10,000 IU IM
- Recombinant hCG 250 μg SC
- Gonadotropin-releasing hormone (GnRH) agonist 2 mg SC.

Functions of these agents are as follows:
- Cellular and nuclear maturation for final meiotic resumption after sperm entry
- Follicular changes for follicular rupture and ovulation
- Induce luteinization in the granulosa cells of the follicle.

Side Effects

They have the potential to precipitate mild to severe OHSS if given in patients with hyperstimulated ovaries.

Adjuvant Drugs to Prevent Premature Luteinizing Hormone Surge with Gonadotropin Therapy

- GnRH agonists in combination with hMG and/or FSH (long, short, or ultrashort protocol)
- GnRH antagonists in combination with hMG and/or FSH (fixed or variable protocol; single- or multiple-dose protocol).

Though LH surge is an absolute requirement for luteinization, final maturation of the oocyte and follicle rupture but a premature LH surge can occur in natural cycle[4,5] and in 25–30% of stimulated cycles resulting in premature luteinization of follicle or early rupture of follicle so that the exact time of ovulation is missed resulting in treatment failures in timed intercourse and IUI cycle.[6,7] A premature LH surge is defined as premature rise of LH (>10 IU/L) accompanied by a simultaneous rise in progesterone levels (>1 mg/L).[6]

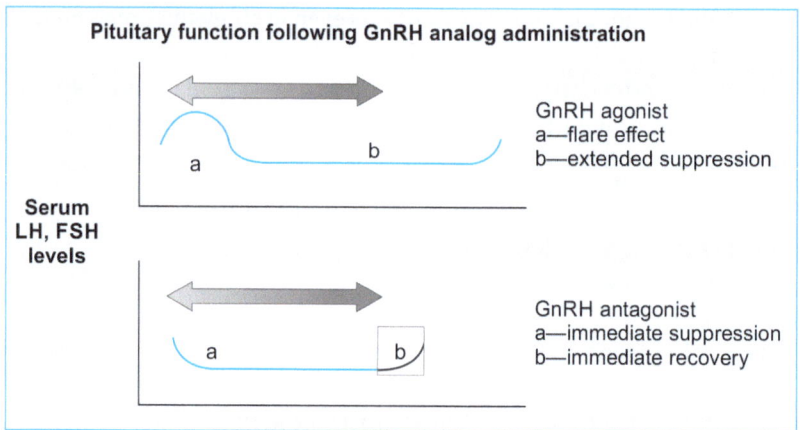

Fig. 8: Pituitary function following gonadotropin-releasing hormone (GnRH) analogs' administration. (FSH: follicle-stimulating hormone; LH: luteinizing hormone)

Whether the use of GnRH agonist or antagonist in IUI cycles is cost effective and helps in improving the outcome needs to be decided.

Moreover, when IUI is done with gonadotropins, the response may vary, ranging from no response to hyper-response (more than four follicles of >12 mm developed). If hyper-response occurs, where follicular recruitment is excessive, a decision must be made to either cancel the cycle or allow the multiple follicles to mature and thus risk the incidence of multiple pregnancy and OHSS or convert it into an IVF cycle.

Gonadotropin-releasing hormone antagonists have the advantage over GnRH agonists as they could be added later in the cycle. The GnRH agonist results in an initial flare followed by extended suppression while antagonist results in immediate suppression and recovery **(Fig. 8)**.

GnRH Agonists in Ovarian Stimulation for Intrauterine Insemination

There seems to be no role for GnRH agonists in IUI programs as they increase the cost as the dose of gonadotropins is increased tremendously. Its use also increases the incidence of multiple pregnancy without increasing the probability of conception. Thus, the use of GnRH agonists with gonadotropins should be carefully considered in an IUI program.[7]

GnRH Antagonists in Ovarian Stimulation for Intrauterine Insemination

When GnRH antagonists are used for ovarian stimulation in combination with IUI[8,9] there may be a small increase in probability of pregnancy. In addition, they may be helpful in cycle programming and avoidance of inseminations during weekends.

Conversion of high-response gonadotropin-IUI cycles to "rescue" IVF using a GnRH antagonist is a cost-effective strategy that produces better results than regular IVF with relatively minimal morbidity, and shorter duration to achieve pregnancy. Implantation and ongoing clinical pregnancy rates tend to be higher than those from hyper-responder regular IVF patients. Whether or not GnRH antagonists should be used regularly in IUI programs needs to be determined in future trials.[7]

■ CONCLUSION

Anovulation is one of the most common causes of reproductive failure in subfertile and infertile couples. In the absence of other significant causes of infertility, successful ovulation induction often will restore normal fertility. CC has been proven to be the best initial treatment in majority of anovulatory infertile women.

Gonadotropin therapy is generally used in CC-resistant patients and in those patients who fail to conceive after repeated courses of CC[10] and those who are for ART.

The aim of ovulation induction with gonadotropins is to find the threshold dose of FSH required to develop a single preovulatory follicle and to avoid multifollicular recruitment[11,12] for non-ART cycles. As the ovarian threshold for FSH response varies among individuals,[12] "step-up protocols" are safest.[13,14]

Individualized protocols selected on evaluation of body mass index (BMI), AFC, AMH, and ovarian response in the preceding CC and gonadotropin cycle reduce the duration of treatment, the amount of gonadotropins administered, the associated risks of cycle-to-cycle variability, multifollicular development, OHSS, and multiple pregnancy. This helps in reducing the complexity and cost while improving the success rate.

Gonadotropin-releasing hormone antagonists may have a role in ovarian stimulation for IUI, but the use of GnRH agonists does not improve the outcome in IUI cycles.

Before treatment with gonadotropins, investigations to rule out other abnormalities such as thyroid function and hyperprolactinemia, and tubal pathology by hysterosalpingography (HSG) should be found out.

Our aim is to use the right drugs after proper evaluation, investigations, and at a proper time. If a patient has a normal ovarian reserve, determining the potential cause of the ovulatory defect is mandatory. In the presence of obesity and chronic anovulation, polycystic ovary syndrome (PCOS), and elevated androgen levels or hyperinsulinemia, the ovulation induction protocols need to be individualized and carefully monitored so that hyper-response does not take place. Patients with diminished ovarian reserve (DOR) also require modification of conventional protocols, but are usually associated with poor prognosis.

> **KEY MESSAGES**
> - Endocrine milieu in women with polycystic ovaries, which may make ovarian stimulation difficult and also increase risk of OHSS.
> - Anti-estrogens appear to be cost effective in IUI programs, although less effective compared to GT.
> - When GT used—given on daily basis.
> - Low-dose protocols do not differ significantly in success, when compared to high dose, which increase risk of multiples and OHSS.
> - No role for GnRH-agonists in IUI programs as they increase costs and risk of MP and OHSS.
> - No difference in the probability of conception whether one uses urinary or Rec GT.
> - Role of GnRH-antagonists in mild COS/IUI programs needs to be determined.
> - Both letrozole and CC have similar results, but letrozole is the first drug of choice.
> - Determinant of success of therapy in women with PCOS depends on presence or absence of obesity, degree of hyperinsulinemia and concentration of circulatory LH.

■ REFERENCES

1. Hillier SG. Paracrine support of ovarian stimulation. Mol Hum Reprod. 2009;15:843-50.
2. Hendriks DJ, Mol BW, Bancsi LF, Te Velde ER, Broekmans FJ. Antral follicle count in the prediction of poor ovarian response and pregnancy after in vitro fertilization: a meta-analysis and comparison with basal follicle-stimulating hormone level. Fertil Steril. 2005;83:291-301.
3. Macklon NS, Stouffer RL, Giudice LC, Fauser BC. The science behind 25 years of ovarian stimulation for in vitro fertilization. Endocr Rev. 2006;27(2):170-207.
4. Klein NA, Harper AJ, Houmard BS, Sluss PM, Soules MR. Is the short follicular phase in older women secondary to advanced or accelerated dominant follicle development? J Clin Endocrinol Metab. 2002;87:5746-50.
5. de Koning CH, McDonnell J, Themmen AP, de Jong FH, Homburg R, Lambalk CB. The endocrine and follicular growth dynamics throughout the menstrual cycle in women with consistently or variably elevated early follicular phase FSH compared with controls. Hum Reprod. 2008;23:1416-23.
6. Lambalk CB, Leader A, Olivennes F, Fluker MR, Andersen AN, Ingerslev J, et al. Treatment with the GnRH antagonist ganirelix prevents premature LH rises and luteinisation in stimulated intrauterine insemination: results of a double-blind, placebo-controlled, multicentre trial. Hum Reprod. 2006;21:632-9.
7. Cantineau AE, Cohlen BJ, Heineman MJ. Ovarian stimulation protocols (anti-oestrogens, gonadotrophins with and without GnRH agonists/antagonists) for intrauterine insemination (IUI) in women with sub fertility (Review). Cochrane Database Syst Rev. 2007;(2):CD005356.
8. Ragni G, Vegetti W, Baroni E, Colombo M, Arnoldi M, Lombroso G, et al. Comparison of luteal phase profile in gonadotropin stimulated cycles with or without a gonadotropin-releasing hormone antagonist. Hum Reprod. 2001;16:2258-62.
9. Gomez-Palomares JL, Julia B, Acevedo-Martin B, Martinez-Burgos M, Hernandez ER, Ricciarelli E. Timing ovulation for intrauterine insemination with a GnRH antagonist. Hum Reprod. 2005;20,368-72.

10. Clark JH, Markaverich BM. The agonistic-antagonistic properties of clomiphene: a review. Pharmacol Ther. 1982;15:467-519.
11. Van Campenhout J, Borreman E, Wyman H, Antaki A. Induction of ovulation with cisclomiphene. Am J Obstet Gynecol. 1973;115:321-7.
12. Young SL, Opsahl MS, Fritz MA. Serum concentrations of enclomiphene and zuclomiphene across consecutive cycles of clomiphene citrate therapy in anovulatory infertile women. Fertil Steril. 1999;71:639-44.
13. Kerin JF, Liu JH, Phillipou G, Yen SS. Evidence for a hypothalamic site of action of clomiphene citrate in women. J Clin Endocrinol Metab. 1985;61:265-8.
14. Rebar R, Judd HL, Yen SSC, Rakoff J, VandenBerg G, Naftolin F. Characterization of the inappropriate gonadotropin secretion in polycystic ovary syndrome. J Clin Invest. 1976;57:1320-9.

Chapter 5

Can Ovarian Response be Improved in Women with Low Ovarian Reserve?

Pratik Tambe

■ BACKGROUND

Millions of in vitro fertilization (IVF)/intracytoplasmic sperm injection (ICSI) cycles take place every year around the world since the technique was perfected in the 1980s. There is an explosive growth in the number of cycles being performed with IVF clinic numbers increasing exponentially in countries such as India. Ovarian stimulation is a key principle of an IVF/ICSI cycle, helping to increase the number of follicles and oocytes to ensure the formation of a good number of embryos which can be transferred to achieve a good clinical pregnancy rate (CPR) and live birth rate (LBR).[1]

Unfortunately, human reproduction is not an exact science and the live birth per mature oocyte is <5%. The number of oocytes required to achieve a successful live birth is also directly proportional to maternal age, reflecting the fact that oocyte quality diminishes with age. The presence of an unexpected poor ovarian response (POR) to gonadotropin stimulation is more frequent and has grown over the past decade in all age groups, resulting in low CPR and LBR.[2,3]

▌EUROPEAN SOCIETY OF HUMAN REPRODUCTION AND EMBRYOLOGY BOLOGNA CONSENSUS[4]

An ovarian response can be defined as POR when at least two of the following three criteria are present:
1. Advanced female age (≥40 years)
2. A previous POR (≤3 oocytes retrieved or cycle canceled)
3. An abnormal ovarian reserve test (ORT) [antral follicle count (AFC) <5 follicles or anti-Müllerian hormone (AMH) <0.5 ng/mL] or in the absence of the above criteria two previous PORs following maximal stimulation.

There are plenty of published studies in the medical literature which confirm that women identified as having a POR by the Bologna criteria exhibit a low CPR and LBR.[5,6]

POSEIDON CLASSIFICATION[7]

However, there is a lot of heterogeneity within the Bologna criteria. In order to be able to better predict the ovarian response and to devise tailor-made strategies for such patients, the Patient-Oriented Strategies Encompassing IndividualizeD Oocyte Number (POSEIDON) classification was proposed. In simple terms, it classifies women both qualitatively and quantitatively giving us a more detailed stratification allowing individualization of treatment and helping to maximize LBR.

According to the POSEIDON criteria, there are four distinct groups of low-prognosis patients, as given in **Box 1**.

A poor response in groups 1 and 2 patients may be owing to insufficient gonadotropin dosage or there may be genetic polymorphism in follicle-stimulating hormone (FSH) or luteinizing hormone (LH) receptors. There are reports in the literature that polymorphisms lead to higher FSH consumption. Supplementation with recombinant luteinizing hormone (rLH) has been suggested to increase the oocyte quality and implantation rates in these groups of patients.

Cumulative Live Birth Rate

As noted earlier, the number of oocytes retrieved and their quality are important determinants of success in IVF cycles. The cumulative live birth rate (CLBR) increases in direct proportion to the number of oocytes retrieved. When 4–9 oocytes are retrieved, the odds ratio of live birth is 2.5 compared to when 0–3 oocytes are retrieved. When 10–15 oocytes are retrieved, the odds ratio is 3.5 and with >15 oocytes, it is 5.6.[8]

BOX 1: Patient-Oriented Strategies Encompassing IndividualizeD Oocyte Number (POSEIDON) classification.

- *Group 1*: Age <35 years with adequate ovarian reserve parameters (AFC ≥5 or AMH ≥1.2 ng/mL)
  - *Subgroup 1A*: Unexpected poor response <4 oocytes retrieved
  - *Subgroup 1B*: Suboptimal response 4–9 oocytes retrieved
- *Group 2*: Age ≥35 years with adequate ovarian reserve parameters (AFC >5 or AMH ≥1.2 ng/mL)
  - *Subgroup 2A*: Unexpected poor response <4 oocytes retrieved
  - *Subgroup 2B*: Suboptimal response 4–9 oocytes retrieved
- *Group 3*: Age <35 years with poor ovarian reserve parameters (AFC <5 or AMH <1.2 ng/mL)
- *Group 4*: Age ≥ 35 years with poor ovarian reserve parameters (AFC <5 or AMH <1.2 ng/mL)

(AFC: antral follicle count; AMH: anti-Müllerian hormone)

Overview of Management

Instead of using the long agonist or short protocol, a gonadotropin-releasing hormone (GnRH) antagonist protocol has been proposed with a view to avoid suppressing innate FSH levels in the early stages of the cycle when follicular recruitment takes place. Some randomized controlled trials (RCTs) have shown similar outcomes between both these protocols. Hence, the antagonist protocol, which is more patient-friendly, requires lesser injections, is more cost-effective, and offers lower FSH consumption per started cycle, would probably be the preferred route.[9,10]

A large RCT comparing mild stimulation with GnRH antagonists compared to a long agonist protocol with conventional stimulation demonstrated an ongoing pregnancy rate of 12.8% (former) versus 13.6% (latter), respectively. The duration of stimulation and consumption of gonadotropin were lower, as expected.[11]

Increasing the gonadotropin dose beyond a particular amount (no difference between 300 and 450 vs. 600 IU) does not yield more follicles or oocytes since the antral follicle numbers are low in these patients. Some newer protocols currently being studied in these women include double ovarian stimulation in the same cycle, i.e., follicular followed by luteal phase stimulation. This may help by increasing available embryos for pooling and, later, segmented embryo transfer.[12]

Some trials have focused on supplementation with recombinant human growth hormone (rhGH) and rLH. Pretreatment with androgens including dehydroepiandrosterone (DHEA), transdermal testosterone, L-arginine, and pyridostigmine are promising though we need more trials with larger numbers before we can make a universal recommendation. Dual trigger administration of GnRH agonist + human chorionic gonadotropin (hCG) may improve the number and maturity of oocytes retrieved, but further evidence is still awaited.[13-15]

Luteal Estradiol Priming

This is done via the administration of 4 mg/day of estradiol valerate starting on day 20 of the previous cycle until the onset of menses. Some centers have used 0.1 mg transdermal estradiol patches instead of oral administration of estradiol valerate. This protocol may not increase pregnancy rates but seems to reduce the cycle cancellation rate with similar oocytes retrieved and embryos formed.[16,17]

Double Stimulation/Shanghai Protocol

In this protocol, gonadotropins are combined with antiestrogenic agents such as clomiphene or letrozole. A GnRH agonist trigger combined with ibuprofen is used for the final maturation before oocyte retrieval. Large mature follicles are aspirated, oocytes retrieved, and resultant embryos are cryopreserved.

Luteal gonadotropin stimulation with an antiestrogenic agent with GnRH antagonist is then performed. The triggering is with the GnRH agonist trigger with ibuprofen again. The final step is endometrial preparation for frozen-thawed embryo transfer. The advantage of this protocol is that a larger number of oocytes are retrieved, potentially increasing the number of embryos available for pooling and subsequent transfer.[18]

Aromatase Inhibitors/Letrozole

Letrozole is a well-known oral ovulogen which is used in basic fertility treatment. It is now considered the agent of choice for ovarian stimulation in polycystic ovary syndrome (PCOS). Lately, it has been used in the treatment of poor responders as it decreases estrogen levels, increases androgen levels, and enhances endogenous FSH production. Letrozole in combination with gonadotropins appears to yield good outcomes compared to high-dose gonadotropins alone.[19]

Supplementation Therapy

Dehydroepiandrosterone pretreatment before the index or treatment cycle in a dose of 25 mg thrice daily for 3–6 months appears to improve the number of oocytes, embryos, CPR, and LBR. However, results are inconsistent and other studies do not report any benefit.[20,21]

■ SUGGESTED STRATEGIES FOR GROUPS 1 AND 2

Pretreatment[22]

Androgen pretreatment with DHEA or transdermal testosterone patches for 3–6 months is suggested for these two groups of patients where ORTs are in the normal range. This is especially effective in group 2 patients. These patients have low follicle-oocyte index (FOI; ratio of oocytes retrieved to follicles visualized; typically <50%). Genotype screening— where available— may reveal FSH or LH receptor polymorphisms **(Box 2)**.

BOX 2: Groups 1 and 2 pretreatment protocols.

Pretreatment protocols:
- AFC ≥5 and/or AMH ≥1.2 ng/mL with a history of suboptimal or poor oocyte number after conventional stimulation
- Consider ART calculator and genotype screening
- Consider androgens in selected patients
  (in particular, POSEIDON group 2 with ovarian reserve markers in the lower limits)

(AFC: antral follicle count; AMH: anti-Müllerian hormone; ART: assisted reproductive technology; POSEIDON: Patient-Oriented Strategies Encompassing IndividualizeD Oocyte Number)

TABLE 1: Groups 1 and 2 stimulation strategies.

Stimulation protocols	POSEIDON group 1 (age <35 years)	POSEIDON group 2 (age ≥35 years)
	Increase recombinant FSH dosage: • 50–75 IU, if no variants • 75–150 IU, if FSH-R variants (maximum daily dose of 300 IU)	Recombinant FSH dose of 300 IU daily
		Consider DuoStim approach
	Consider adding rLH 2:1 ratio of rFSH and rLH from the first stimulation day in women who consumed >3,000 IU or with a history of follicular stagnation	POSEIDON group 2 (age 35–39 years)
		rLH 150 IU daily from stimulation day 1 in both agonist and antagonist regimens

(FSH-R: follicle-stimulating hormone receptor; POSEIDON: Patient-Oriented Strategies Encompassing IndividualizeD Oocyte Number; rFSH: recombinant follicle-stimulating hormone; rLH: recombinant luteinizing hormone)

Stimulation Strategies

Consider increasing FSH dosage up to a maximum of 300 IU/day. Addition of rLH in a ratio of 2:1 (FSH:LH) may help some women who have high requirements/FSH consumption, especially if their age is <35 years. For group 2 patients, a DuoStim approach (Shanghai protocol) might be in order. Addition of rLH is recommended for group 2 patients from day 1 of stimulation **(Table 1)**.

Trigger/Retrieval/Transfer Recommendations

A GnRH antagonist cycle with GnRH agonist trigger and frozen embryo transfer (FET) is recommended in group 1 patients. Preimplantation genetic testing for aneuploidy (PGT-A) is ideal in group 2 patients. A single blastocyst transfer strategy yields best results. In group 1, around five oocytes are required for one euploid embryo. In group 2, 10–12 mature oocytes are needed for one euploid embryo **(Box 3)**.

■ SUGGESTED STRATEGIES FOR GROUP 3

Stimulation with the long gonadotropin-releasing hormone agonist (GnRHa) protocol or GnRH antagonist with estradiol or oral contraceptive pill (OCP) pretreatment yields best results. DuoStim may be utilized. Androgens may

BOX 3: Groups 1 and 2 trigger/retrieval/transfer.

Trigger/retrieval:
- Consider antagonist regimen, GnRHa trigger, and elective embryo freezing in cases of AFC >16 and/or AMH >3.36 ng/mL
- Consider preimplantation genetic testing for aneuploidy (PGT-A) in POSEIDON group 2 (in particular, patients aged >38 years)
- Consider single blastocyst embryo transfer

(AFC: antral follicle count; AMH: anti-Müllerian hormone; GnRHa: gonadotropin-releasing hormone agonist; POSEIDON: Patient-Oriented Strategies Encompassing IndividualizeD Oocyte Number)

be beneficial. Stimulation with 300 IU recombinant follicle-stimulating hormone (rFSH) is recommended. A fresh transfer may be performed or oocyte/embryo pooling with staged FET is a good alternative. Around four to five oocytes are necessary to yield one euploid embryo on average.

■ SUGGESTED STRATEGIES FOR GROUP 4

Stimulation with the long GnRHa protocol or GnRH antagonist with estradiol or OCP pretreatment yields best results. DuoStim may be utilized. Androgens may be beneficial. Stimulation with 300 IU rFSH is recommended. Addition of rLH to the stimulation protocol may yield better results. A fresh transfer may be performed or oocyte/embryo pooling with staged FET is a good alternative. Preimplantation genetic screening (PGS) may be offered where available. Oocyte donation is an option where legally permitted. Around 12 oocytes are necessary to yield one euploid embryo on average.

■ META-ANALYSIS

A retrospective meta-analysis published in 2019 evaluated 26,697 IVF cycles and calculated the optimal and conservative CLBR per cycle. In POSEIDON groups 1, 2, 3, and 4, the CLBRs per initiated cycle were 56.0%, 30.1%, 14.7%, and 6.6%, respectively. After three completed cycles, the optimal and conservative CLBR were 83.9% and 66.1%, 53.7% and 37.7%, and 44.2%, 28.0%, 14.2%, and 9.7% in groups 1, 2, 3, and 4, respectively. These figures may be used to counsel patients newly diagnosed as poor responders to provide them with an accurate prognosis as to their chances of conceiving.[23]

■ CONCLUSION

The incidence of women undergoing assisted reproduction who exhibit a POR is increasing. This is defined as <4 oocytes retrieved (suboptimal is 4–9 oocytes) after a conventional stimulation. The Bologna criteria and the newer POSEIDON classification have helped increase our understanding of this entity. Groups 1 and 2 patients respond poorly, either owing to receptor polymorphisms or inadequate responses to standard stimulation dosages.

The primary goal of management in groups 1 and 2 patients is to maximize oocyte yield and achieve at least one euploid embryo for an embryo transfer. Genetic testing for receptor polymorphisms may be offered where available. As per the current literature, there are at least five proven strategies to be considered: (1) Use of recombinant FSH, (2) maximizing the FSH dosage, (3) rLH supplementation, (4) pretreatment with androgens, and (5) DuoStim/Shanghai protocol. Further trials are needed to determine the best strategies for the treatment of patients, but in general, individualized stimulation protocols currently offer the greatest benefit.

KEY MESSAGES

- Bologna criteria, while being a step forward, may still not be perfect due to heterogeneity of subgroups and as specific profiles of abnormal ovarian response (hypo- and sub-optimal) are not included. This classification also did not take into account the age-related aneuploidies.
- So, the POSEIDON classification was suggested which included low prognosis patient with good and poor ovarian reserve.
- Insufficient evidence for most adjuvants to improve outcome.
- Growth hormone may improve outcome by increasing of oocytes retrieved and may result in more transferable embryos.
- Pre-treatment with DHEA/testosterone gel priming/COQ10 may improve CPR.
- Co-treatment with estradiol in previous luteal phase to synchronize follicles is not beneficial.
- CC and letrozole decrease the dose of exogenous GTs, however, have a negative impact on implantation.
- No evidence for any particular COS protocol to improve treatment outcome.
- Though the GnRH agonist protocol yields more oocytes with a higher cumulative LBR as compared to GnRH antagonist protocols, but GnRH-antagonist protocols may reduce treatment burden.
- Increasing dose of FSH does not increase CPR and cumulative LBR. LH seems to increase the number of oocytes retrieved (+0.75) and CPR (+30%).
- Poor responders are not homogeneous for pregnancy prospects.
- Female age and number of oocytes retrieved will modulate the chances for pregnancy in current and subsequent cycles.
- Start stimulation when baseline US shows sufficient number of follicles, and it is better to use a combination of FSH and LH.
- Synchronize the follicle pool with premenstrual estrogen/P4 treatment or long protocol.
- Dual stimulation or pooling when appropriate.
- Use of embryo selection techniques such as transfer at the blastocyst stage, PGT-A, time lapse are still questionable.

■ REFERENCES

1. Roque M, Haahr T, Esteves SC, Humaidan P. The POSEIDON stratification—moving from poor ovarian response to low prognosis. JBRA Assist Reprod. 2021;25(2):282-92.

2. Goldman RH, Racowsky C, Farland LV, Munné S, Ribustello L, Fox JH. Predicting the likelihood of live birth for elective oocyte cryopreservation: a counseling tool for physicians and patients. Hum Reprod. 2017;32:853-9.
3. Humaidan P, Chin W, Rogoff D, D'Hooghe T, Longobardi S, Hubbard J, et al. Efficacy and safety of follitropin alfa/lutropin alfa in ART: a randomized controlled trial in poor ovarian responders. Hum Reprod. 2017;32:544-5.
4. Ferraretti AP, La Marca A, Fauser BC, Tarlatzis B, Nargund G, Gianaroli L, et al. ESHRE consensus on the definition of 'poor response' to ovarian stimulation for in vitro fertilization: the Bologna criteria. Hum Reprod. 2011;26:1616-24.
5. Grisendi V, Mastellari E, La Marca A. Ovarian reserve markers to identify poor responders in the context of POSEIDON classification. Front Endocrinol (Lausanne). 2019;10:281.
6. Bozdag G, Polat M, Yarali I, Yarali H. Live birth rates in various subgroups of poor ovarian responders fulfilling the Bologna criteria. Reprod Biomed Online. 2017;34:639-44.
7. Poseidon Group (Patient-Oriented Strategies Encompassing Individualized Oocyte Number), Alviggi C, Andersen CY, Buehler K, Conforti A, Placido G, et al. A new more detailed stratification of low responders to ovarian stimulation: from a poor ovarian response to a low prognosis concept. Fertil Steril. 2016;105:1452-3.
8. Drakopoulos P, Blockeel C, Stoop D, Camus M, de Vos M, Tournaye H, et al. Estimulação ovariana convencional e transferência de embrião único para FIV/ICSI. Quantos oócitos precisamos para maximizar as taxas cumulativas de nascidos vivos após a utilização de todos os embriões frescos e congelados? Hum Reprod. 2016;31:370-6.
9. Lambalk CB, Banga FR, Huirne JA, Toftager M, Pinborg A, Homburg R, et al. GnRH antagonist versus long agonist protocols in IVF: a systematic review and meta-analysis accounting for patient type. Hum Reprod Update. 2017;23:560-79.
10. Pandian Z, McTavish AR, Aucott L, Hamilton MP, Bhattacharya S. Interventions for 'poor responders' to controlled ovarian hyper stimulation (COH) in in-vitro fertilisation (IVF). Cochrane Database Syst Rev. 2010;(1):CD004379.
11. Youssef MA, van Wely M, Al-Inany H, Madani T, Jahangiri N, Khodabakhshi S, et al. A mild ovarian stimulation strategy in women with poor ovarian reserve undergoing IVF: a multicenter randomized non-inferiority trial. Hum Reprod. 2017;32:112-8.
12. Jin B, Niu Z, Xu B, Chen Q, Zhang A. Comparison of clinical outcomes among dual ovarian stimulation, mild stimulation and luteal phase stimulation protocols in women with poor ovarian response. Gynecol Endocrinol. 2018;34:694.
13. Santi D, Casarini L, Alviggi C, Simoni M. Efficacy of follicle-stimulating hormone (FSH) alone, FSH + luteinizing hormone, human menopausal gonadotropin or FSH + human chorionic gonadotropin on assisted reproductive technology outcomes in the "personalized" medicine era: a meta-analysis. Front Endocrinol (Lausanne). 2017;8:114.
14. Haahr T, Esteves SC, Humaidan P. Individualized controlled ovarian stimulation in expected poor-responders: an update. Reprod Biol Endocrinol. 2018;16:20.
15. Mak SM, Wong WY, Chung HS, Chung PW, Kong GW. Effect of mid-follicular phase recombinant LH versus urinary HCG supplementation in poor ovarian responders undergoing IVF—a prospective double-blinded randomized study. Reprod Biomed Online. 2017;34:258.

16. Reynolds KA, Omurtag KR, Jimenez PT, Rhee JS, Tuuli MG. Cycle cancellation and pregnancy after luteal estradiol priming in women defined as poor responders: a systematic review and meta-analysis. Hum Reprod. 2013;28:2981.
17. Lukaszuk K, Liss J, Kunicki M, Kuczynski W, Pastuszek E, Jakiel G, et al. Estradiol valerate pretreatment in short protocol GnRH-agonist cycles versus combined pretreatment with oral contraceptive pills in long protocol GnRH-agonist cycles: a randomised controlled trial. Biomed Res Int. 2015;2015:628056.
18. Kuang Y, Chen Q, Hong Q, Lyu Q, Ai A, Fu Y, et al. Double stimulations during the follicular and luteal phases of poor responders in IVF/ICSI programmes (Shanghai protocol). Reprod Biomed Online. 2014;29:684.
19. Bastu E, Buyru F, Ozsurmeli M, Demiral I, Dogan M, Yeh J. A randomized, single-blind, prospective trial comparing three different gonadotropin doses with or without addition of letrozole during ovulation stimulation in patients with poor ovarian response. Eur J Obstet Gynecol Reprod Biol. 2016;203:30.
20. Liu Y, Hu L, Fan L, Wang F. Efficacy of dehydroepiandrosterone (DHEA) supplementation for in vitro fertilization and embryo transfer cycles: a systematic review and meta-analysis. Gynecol Endocrinol. 2018;34:178.
21. Narkwichean A, Maalouf W, Campbell BK, Jayaprakasan K. Efficacy of dehydroepiandrosterone to improve ovarian response in women with diminished ovarian reserve: a meta-analysis. Reprod Biol Endocrinol. 2013;11:44.
22. Conforti A, Esteves SC, Cimadomo D, Vaiarelli A, Di Rella F, Ubaldi FM, et al. Manejo de mulheres com uma resposta ovariana inesperada baixa à gonadotrofina. Front Endocrinol (Lausanne). 2019;10:387.
23. Li Y, Li X, Yang X, Cai S, Lu G, Lin G, et al. Cumulative live birth rates in low prognosis patients according to the POSEIDON criteria: an analysis of 26,697 cycles of in vitro fertilization/intracytoplasmic sperm injection. Front Endocrinol (Lausanne). 2019;10:642.

Chapter 6

Adjuvants in Polycystic Ovary Syndrome

Rakhi Singh, Meenu Handa, Madhuri Patil

■ INTRODUCTION

Polycystic ovary syndrome (PCOS) is a common endocrinological problem spanning across all reproductive ages. It affects up to 18% of premenopausal reproductive aged women and is the most common metabolic issue in this age group, depending on the population studied and diagnostic criteria used.[1] PCOS is a very common metabolic problem and affects around 30 obese women and up to 5% of lean women.[2]

Polycystic ovary syndrome is commonly associated with metabolic derangements, cosmetic issues, and altered reproductive, psychological, and sexual functions. Polycystic ovarian disease (PCOD) is multifactorial in origin and is typically characterized by a disproportionate increase in intraovarian androgens, leading to menstrual irregularity, polycystic ovaries, subfertility, and biochemical/clinical hyperandrogenism.[3]

Many studies have noted various etiology contributing to PCOS ranging from genetic causes and environmental contributors to hormonal disturbances characterized in PCOS (along with obesity, ovarian dysfunction, and hypothalamic–pituitary abnormalities).[4] Though insulin resistance (IR) has been undoubtedly regarded as a major contributor to the PCOS etiology, the exact pathophysiology of PCOS is complex and remains unclear till date.[5] The American Diabetes Association has characterized IR as a state of impaired metabolic response to insulin.[6] The main derangement in IR is the impairment of insulin to maintain euglycemia and glucose homeostasis. Impairment of glucose homeostasis includes impaired glucose uptake, glycogen synthesis, and inhibition of lipolysis, resulting in pancreas to oversecrete insulin to achieve euglycemia.[7] Hyperinsulinemia thus caused due to IR in PCOS women in turn leads to dysregulation in lipid metabolism, deranging protein synthesis and androgen production.[8] We now understand that IR is often the early hormonal disturbance in the disease progression of diabetes mellitus seen later in life and also predisposes PCOS women to cardiovascular diseases. Hence, it is important to treat women having IR. In 2012, the National Institutes of Health (NIH) consensus workshop on

PCOS endorsed the Rotterdam criteria as the definitive diagnostic criteria and recommended that all studies include analyses by reproductive PCOS phenotype.[9] In 2018, recommendations from the international evidence-based guideline for the assessment and management of PCOS clearly reemphasized to use Rotterdam criteria for diagnosing PCOS and to assess glycemic status at baseline in all women with PCOS due to IR.[10] It has been recommended to evaluate glycemic status in PCOS women using glycated hemoglobin (HbA1c) or fasting glucose.

■ METFORMIN

Over the past few decades, metformin has been the cornerstone in the treatment for PCOS women diagnosed to have IR or impaired glucose tolerance. IR has been found in clamp studies in 75% of lean women and 95% of overweight women.[10,11] Metformin is a biguanide working on the liver and its main action is to inhibit hepatic gluconeogenesis. It diminishes the fatty acid production by inhibiting the enzyme acetyl-CoA carboxylase. Metformin also works on skeletal muscle and inhibits the production of lipids as well as has peripheral action on adipose tissues by increasing glucose uptake. It has also been shown to improve insulin receptor activity and in turn aids in reducing insulin levels.[12] International Diabetes Federation recommends the use of metformin for diabetes prevention in all those patients where lifestyle modifications have failed to achieve a euglycemic state.[13] PCOS women have increased IR and a high-risk of type 2 diabetes mellitus (DM2), and the risk is even higher when other risk factors preexist such as excess weight, family history of DM2, metabolic syndrome, or prediabetes.[14]

As per 2018 recommendations from the international evidence-based guideline for the assessment and management of PCOS, the following key points were suggested regarding use of metformin:[10]
- Along with lifestyle modifications, metformin may be recommended in PCOS women and in overweight PCOS [body mass index (BMI) ≥ 25 kg/m^2] for the treatment of weight, hormonal and metabolic outcomes.
- Metformin, in addition to lifestyle, could be considered in adolescents with a clear diagnosis of PCOS or with symptoms of PCOS before the diagnosis is made.
- Metformin may offer greater benefit in high metabolic risk groups, including those with diabetes risk factors, impaired glucose tolerance, or high-risk ethnic groups.
- To minimize the side effects of metformin, it is advisable to start with low dose of 500 mg with steady increments 1–2 weekly and extended-release preparations to minimize side effects.
- Dose-dependent common adverse effects such as gastrointestinal disturbances are generally self-limiting.

- Metformin use appears safe long term, based on use in other populations; however, ongoing requirement needs to be considered and its use may be associated with low vitamin B_{12} level.

■ MYOINOSITOL

Myoinositol (MI) is one stereoisomer of a C_6 sugar alcohol that belongs to the inositol family.[15] It is also the precursor of inositol triphosphate and is also known to act as an intracellular second messenger. MI regulates many hormones such as thyroid-stimulating hormone (TSH), follicle-stimulating hormone (FSH), and insulin.[16] Studies suggested MI and D-chiro-inositol (DCI), another stereoisomeric form of inositol, to play a crucial role in the complex metabolic regulations concurring with IR. It was seen that MI-derived phosphatidylinositol-3,4,5-trisphosphate (PIP3) enhances glucose transport inside the cells through the stimulation of glucose transporter type 4 (GLUT4) translocation to the cell membrane. Through an intricate pathway, PIP3 downregulated the release of free fatty acids from adipose tissues.[17] MI along with DCI improved the IR and was found to be an important adjunct in the treatment of PCOS. Another important area where MI is seen to be beneficial is increasing sex hormone-binding globulin (SHBG). SHBG is a protein that binds to testosterone, making it unavailable to target tissues. The higher the levels of SHBG, the lower the bioavailability of testosterone. It thus minimizes the hyperandrogenic features characterized in IR caused by PCOS. Furthermore, SHBG is noted in many studies as a valuable marker of IR in PCOS. In a recent meta-analysis, it was shown that the increase in serum SHBG is noted only in those trials which supplemented inositol(s) for at least 24 weeks.[18] It was also shown in this meta-analysis that there is a beneficial effect of administration of DCI along with MI as it is seen that IR patients with PCOS have low endogenous DCI synthesis and its excessive urinary excretion. At the same time, it was noted that DCI supplementation alone is not found to be effective and in fact increasing the dosage of DCI alone can worsen the oocyte quality and ovarian response.[19] There is ample evidence to suggest the beneficial effect exerted by MI and DCI combined at 40:1 ratio in PCOS patients.[20]

■ VITAMIN D

Last few decades, it has been noted that vitamin D does play a crucial role apart from calcium and bone homeostasis. Pancreatic beta cells, immune cells, and also the reproductive organs showed evidence of presence of vitamin D receptors and the enzyme 1 alpha-hydroxylase.[21] Many studies have indicated the role of vitamin D in the etiopathogenesis of PCOS through gene transcription and on glucose homeostasis through direct as well as indirect ways.[22] Vitamin D exerts its direct effect through vitamin D receptors present on the pancreatic beta cells and through the presence of vitamin D—response element present on the human insulin promoter gene.[23] One of the largest epidemiological studies showed a significant association between vitamin D status and metabolic disturbances in patients with PCOS. It was shown that PCOS women had significantly lower serum 25-hydroxyvitamin D [25(OH)D] compared to fertile controls. A compromised vitamin D status in PCOS women is associated with a higher HOMA-IR (homeostatic model assessment for insulin resistance) and an unfavorable lipid profile.[24]

■ N-ACETYLCYSTEINE

N-acetylcysteine (NAC) increases the cellular levels of antioxidant and reduces glutathione at higher doses. NAC has been seen to improve insulin receptor activity and, in turn, improves insulin secretion during glucose metabolism. Thus, it helps to decrease hyperinsulinemia and that, in turns, leads to significant drop in free androgens. It helps in decreasing the androgen in the ovarian microenvironment and improves the follicular response in PCOS women undergoing fertility treatment.[25] In a recent systemic review and meta-analysis, it was shown that in PCOS women undergoing fertility treatment when given NAC as an adjunct, significant pregnancy and ovulation rate result as compared to placebo.[26]

■ CHROMIUM POLY-NICOTINATE

Chromium poly-nicotinate binds to niacin also know as vitamin B3 and provides a biologically active form of chromium, and makes it easier for the body to absorb. It is an active component of glucose tolerance factor which is responsible for binding insulin to cell membrane receptor sites and thus improves insulin sensitivity and stimulates the metabolism of sugar, fat and cholesterol.

■ MELATONIN

It is the hormone of pineal gland, maintain normal circadian rhythms, govern release of pituitary gonadotropins. Melatonin receptors have been identified in anterior pituitary and ovary also. It is involved in follicular development, ovulation, oocyte maturation, and luteal function. Melatonin deficiency seems to be involved in pathophysiology of PCOS and thus it can be used as an adjuvant in PCOS. It is also a powerful free radical scavenger and has broad-spectrum antioxidant property. On administration, it is taken up into the follicular fluid from the blood. Reactive oxygen species (ROS) produced within the follicles, especially during the ovulation process, were scavenged by melatonin, and reduced oxidative stress involved in oocyte maturation and embryo development. It also increases intrafollicular melatonin concentrations and reduces intrafollicular oxidative damage. These mechanism can improve oocyte quality and may improve the pregnancy rates. But despite these advantages and antioxidant action of Melatonin as per recent meta-analysis, there is no clarity regarding benefit of adding melatonin in all PCOS women.

L-METHYL FOLATE

L-Methyl folate is a natural, active form of folic acid used at the cellular level for DNA reproduction and the regulation of homocysteine. It reduces homocysteine levels and prevents cardiovascular risk factors associated with PCOS. Its un-methylated form, folic acid (vitamin B_9), is a synthetic form of folate found in nutritional supplements.

CO-ENZYME 10 (COQ10)

CoQ10 seems to be a promising adjuvant to oral ovulatory agents such as CC effective, inexpensive and safe for stimulating follicular development in CC-resistant PCOS and can be tried successfully before a more complicated treatment such as GTs and laparoscopic ovarian drilling.

CONCLUSION

An adjuvant is a substance that enhances the pharmacological effect of a drug. Though the evidence is limited on the use of adjuvants. It can be used in PCOS as PCOS is an enigma the pathophysiology not fully understood, and the treatment is directed at symptoms and not at syndrome. A well-designed and adequately powered RCT is desired to prove the efficacy of these adjuvants in PCOS. Of all the adjuvants described metformin definitely has a role in management of PCOS.

KEY MESSAGES

- Off-label prescription of adjuvants for the treatment of PCOS is widespread.
- In the field of reproductive medicine, it is common for an innovative practice to become widely used before demonstration of its efficacy.
- Patients with infertility are particularly vulnerable to trying new treatments in hopes of conceiving.
- Good medical practice dictates that the physician keep the best interest of their patients in mind and counsel patients appropriately about the best evidence available and potential adverse effects of the treatments prescribed.
- One needs to balance the benefits with the evidence when using adjuvants in PCOS.
- Metformin alone may be beneficial over placebo for LBR, although the quality of evidence was low. Results differed by BMI, emphasizing the importance of stratifying results by BMI.
- Inositols induces nuclear and cytoplasmic oocyte maturation and promotes embryo development but there is no data on its effects on PR and LBRs.

Contd...

Contd...

- Vitamin D binds to vitamin D receptor activates peroxisome proliferator activator receptor-δ (PPAR-δ) and stimulates the expression of insulin receptor thus enhances insulin-mediated glucose transport.
- N-acetyl-cysteine could improve the insulin sensitivity and hormonal profile therefore might be beneficial in improving ovarian response to ovarian stimulation and IVF outcomes.
- Melatonin due to its antioxidant capacity may improve oocyte quality and pregnancy rates but the evidence is very sparse.
- Data on use of chromium polynicotinate and L-methyl folate is very limited.

■ REFERENCES

1. March WA, Moore VM, Willson KJ, Phillips DI, Norman RJ, Davies MJ. The prevalence of polycystic ovary syndrome in a community sample assessed under contrasting diagnostic criteria. Hum Reprod. 2010;25:544-51.
2. Alvarez-Blasco F, Botella-Carretero JI, San Millán JL, Escobar-Morreale HF. Prevalence and characteristics of the polycystic ovary syndrome in overweight and obese women. Arch Intern Med. 2006;166:2081-6.
3. Nasr A. Effect of N-acetyl-cysteine after ovarian drilling in clomiphene citrate-resistant PCOS women: a pilot study. Reprod Biomed Online. 2010;20(3):403-9.
4. Legro RS, Strauss JF. Molecular progress in infertility: polycystic ovary syndrome. Fertil Steril 2002;78:569-76.
5. Legro RS, Castracane VD, Kauffman RP. Detecting insulin resistance in polycystic ovary syndrome: purposes and pitfalls. Obstet Gynecol Surv. 2004;59:141-54.
6. Consensus Development Conference on Insulin Resistance. 5-6 November 1997. American Diabetes Association. Diabetes Care. 1998;21:310-4.
7. Diamanti-Kandarakis E, Dunaif A. Insulin resistance and the polycystic ovary syndrome revisited: an update on mechanisms and implications. Endocr Rev. 2012;33:981-1030.
8. Teede H, Deeks A, Moran L. Polycystic ovary syndrome: a complex condition with psychological, reproductive and metabolic manifestations that impacts on health across the lifespan. BMC Med. 2010;8:41.
9. National Institutes of Health. (2012). Polycystic ovary syndrome.
10. Teede HJ, Misso ML, Costello MF, Dokras A, Laven J, Moran L, et al. Recommendations from the international evidence-based guideline for the assessment and management of polycystic ovary syndrome. Fertil Steril. 2018;110:364-79.
11. Stepto NK, Cassar S, Joham AE, Hutchison SK, Harrison CL, Goldstein RF, et al. Women with polycystic ovary syndrome have intrinsic insulin resistance on euglycaemic-hyperinsulaemic clamp. Hum Reprod. 2013;28(3):777-84.
12. De Leo V, Musacchio MC, Palermo V, Di Sabatino A, Morgante G, Petraglia F. Polycystic ovary syndrome and metabolic comorbidities: therapeutic options. Drugs Today (Barc). 2009;45:763-75.
13. Meyer C, McGrath BP, Teede HJ. Effects of medical therapy on insulin resistance and the cardiovascular system in polycystic ovary syndrome. Diabetes Care. 2007;30:471-8.

14. Teede HJ, Hutchison SK, Zoungas S. The management of insulin resistance in polycystic ovary syndrome. Trends Endocrinol Metab. 2007;18:273-9.
15. Bizzarri M, Fuso A, Dinicola S, Cucina A, Bevilacqua A. Pharmacodynamics and pharmacokinetics of inositol(s) in health and disease. Expert Opin Drug Metab Toxicol. 2016;12:1181-96.
16. Di Paolo G, De Camilli P. Phosphoinositides in cell regulation and membrane dynamics. Nature. 2006;443:651-7.
17. Paul C, Laganà AS, Maniglio P, Triolo O, Brady DM. Inositol's and other nutraceuticals' synergistic actions counteract insulin resistance in polycystic ovarian syndrome and metabolic syndrome: state-of-the-art and future perspectives. Gynecol Endocrinol. 2016;32:431-8.
18. Unfer V, Facchinetti F, Orrù B, Giordani B, Nestler J. Myo-inositol effects in women with PCOS: a meta-analysis of randomized controlled trials. Endocr Connect. 2017;6:647-58.
19. Isabella R, Raffone E. CONCERN: does ovary need d-chiro-inositol? J Ovarian Res. 2012;5:14.
20. Benelli E, Del Ghianda S, Di Cosmo C, Tonacchera M. A combined therapy with myo-inositol and d-chiro-inositol improves endocrine parameters and insulin resistance in PCOS young overweight women. Int J Endocrinol. 2016;2016:3204083.
21. Bland R, Markovic D, Hills CE, Hughes SV, Chan SLF, Squires PE, et al. Expression of 25-hydroxyvitamin D3-1alpha-hydroxylase in pancreatic islets. J Steroid Biochem Mol Biol. 2004;89-90(1-5):121-5
22. Mahmoudi T. Genetic variation in the vitamin D receptor and polycystic ovary syndrome risk. Fertil Steril. 2009;92(4):1381-3.
23. Maestro B, Dávila N, Carranza MC, Calle C. Identification of a vitamin D response element in the human insulin receptor gene promoter. J Steroid Biochem Mol Biol. 2003;84(2-3):223-30.
24. Krul-Poel YHM, Koenders PP, Steegers-Theunissen RP, Ten Boekel E, Wee MMT, Louwers Y, et al. Vitamin D and metabolic disturbances in polycystic ovary syndrome (PCOS): a cross-sectional study. PLoS One. 2018;13:e0204748.
25. Elnashar A, Fahmy M, Mansour A, Ibrahim K. N-acetyl cysteine vs. metformin in treatment of clomiphene citrate-resistant polycystic ovary syndrome: a prospective randomized controlled study. Fertil Steril. 2007;88(2):406-9.
26. Thakker D, Raval A, Patel I, Walia R. N-Acetylcysteine for polycystic ovary syndrome: a systematic review and meta-analysis of randomized controlled clinical trials. Obstet Gynecol Int. 2015;2015:817849.

Chapter 7

Optimizing Ovarian Stimulation for Assisted Reproductive Technology Outcomes in Women with Advanced Endometriosis

Shalini Gainder, Parul Kotdawala

■ INTRODUCTION

Endometriosis is a disease affecting women in the reproductive age, where there is presence of endometrial tissue outside the uterine cavity. It has potential to impact the reproductive performance of women and may compromise their fertility potential.[1] About 25–50% of infertile patients are diagnosed to have endometriosis.[2] As many as 30–50% women with endometriosis report difficulties attempting conception.[2] Infertility in these women may be caused by various reasons directly due to anatomical distortions as a result of scarring and adhesions or due to formation of endometrioma in the ovary affecting the ovulation and by decreasing ovarian reserve. It disturbs the process of folliculogenesis and alters the milieu of the pelvic cavity by inflammatory response of the disease, as well as associated immunological factors of the disease.[3,4] Sometimes, there are associated leiomyomas or adenomyosis present in the uterus, which may reduce her fertility. There is an association of endometriosis with uterine malformation and adenomyosis, which may interfere the implantation and nidation of the fertilized embryo.

The disease may variably impact a woman and should be graded according to standardized classification used for endometriosis for documentation after surgical procedure and for research and publication. The European Society of Human Reproduction and Embryology (ESHRE) 2022 recommends using endometriosis fertility index (EFI), which includes scores from the American Society for Reproductive Medicine (ASRM) system.[5] This classification is a combination of using surgical stage of the disease and medical history of the women such as her age, duration of infertility, and prior reproductive performance in determining her probability of achieving a conception.[5-8]

Once a woman is diagnosed to have endometriosis, there is a concern of her future fertility, and this depends largely on the ovarian reserve of the woman, the stage of disease—its progression, and the treatment offered. ESHRE and various available literatures suggest that in a woman desiring conception, controlled ovarian stimulation should be offered rather than watchful expectancy or no treatment. The aim of this write-up based on the available evidence is to update regarding ovarian stimulation in women desiring fertility, especially in cases of advanced endometriosis.

Factors Impacting the Ovarian Response in Endometriosis

- The anti-Müllerian hormone (AMH) level of the patient predicting the ovarian reserve
- The presence of endometrioma
- The presence of peritubal adhesions will affect only in "controlled ovarian stimulation" as this may increase failure of follicle to rupture ending in luteinized unruptured follicle
- The location of ovary and its adhesion may impact the follicle retrieval by accounting for difficult retrieval due to difficult placement
- The absence of ovary in cases of previous surgery.

Serum Anti-Müllerian Hormone Correlation in Endometriosis

The ovarian involvement in endometriosis impacts the ovarian reserve and its ability to ovulate or respond to controlled ovarian stimulation. The presence of endometrioma seems to impact the ovarian reserve as well as the removal of the same even in best surgical hands.[9,10] AMH levels may show some improvement after 12 months of surgery. The factors that directly impact the levels are bilateral cysts, the stage of the disease, and the size of endometrioma.[11,12] The AMH level may be impacted by the endometrioma of >5 cm, with women having lower AMH if both ovaries showed endometrioma compared to women with unilateral endometrioma. It has been seen that women with smaller endometrioma also show decreased ovarian reserve compared to matched controls without the disease.[12,13] Women with endometriosis undergoing in vitro fertilization (IVF) have lower AMH levels compared with age-matched controls without endometriosis.[14] Even in women with stage I and II disease, the serum AMH levels were found lower in a small case–control study; however, this result has not been supported by other studies.[15] Mere presence of endometrioma can lower AMH even without a surgery, and since this is not observed in women with simple cyst(s), it is obvious that the endometriosis does lead to suppressive effect on AMH and ovarian reserve.[12] In a few studies, it has been observed that the presence of endometrioma may paradoxically lead to an elevated level of AMH. This happens due to the presence of vascular endothelial growth factor (VEGF) levels, which increases the neovascularization and therefore may not predict the true response to gonadotropins.[16,17] The increased VEGF levels in women with endometriosis have been proven in many previous studies.[18,19]

Ovarian Response in Relation to Anti-Müllerian Hormone Levels

The antral follicle count is used to predict the ovarian reserve in women needing ovarian stimulation for assisted reproductive technology (ART) and predict response to the treatment, whereas in these women, there is a complete anatomical distortion due to the presence of endometrioma either prior to surgery or due to recurrence of the disease despite surgery. This makes it difficult to assess the ovarian reserve by transvaginal ultrasonography. Sometimes, the ovaries are placed outside the visual field of the probe used due to associated adenomyosis or fibroid. All these factors compromise the assessment of ovary.

The AMH levels are low in most women with endometriosis and predict the poor response to the gonadotropins. There are other factors that may affect the ovarian response in cases of endometriosis such as presence of fibrosis, atretic follicles, loss of cortex-specific stroma, and decreased density of antral follicles leading to overall lower AMH values. Over the last two decades, with rising cases of laparoscopic approach and heavy reliance on electrocautery to achieve hemostasis during lap surgery in endometriosis, a higher rate of thermal damage due to deep and lateral spread in the ovarian tissues led to postoperative depletion of ovarian reserve in young women desiring fertility. Now with the better understanding of electrosurgical devices, precisely acting energy sources, use of laser, and increase in expertise, these adverse effects are relatively controlled.

The ESHRE has recently published its position statement about endometriosis and fertility, wherein it recommends limited use of surgery prior to ART.[20] This has changed the practice of performing surgery, and fewer women are advised surgery for endometriosis in subfertility patients:
- Women with visible ovarian anatomy distortion due to the presence of endometriosis
- Difficult oocyte access for ART
- Presence of associated myoma (to correct cavity shape)
- Combined ovarian and uterine surgeries if there is concomitant presence of uterine anomaly or hydrosalpinx or hematosalpinx, which may prompt the fertility expert to consider surgical correction prior to ART.

PREPARING FOR ASSISTED REPRODUCTIVE TECHNOLOGY IN WOMEN WITH SEVERE ENDOMETRIOSIS

Role of Ovarian Suppression Before Assisted Reproductive Technology

It is a well-established fact that endometriosis responds well to the various progesterone preparations used for medical management of the disease.

The other drugs used in disease suppression are combined estrogen progesterone pills used in young women of reproductive age. The gonadotropin releasing hormone (GnRH) agonists also cause marked suppression, and this has been used in various studies in women needing treatment of infertility and prior to ART.

Recent data and evidence have shifted toward not using any suppressive drug in women desiring pregnancy as the evidence review by Cochrane database failed to demonstrate significant difference in pregnancy outcome between women who received suppression and women who were not suppressed.[21]

Based on this evidence, the ESHRE 2022 guideline[20] has made a strong recommendation against the use of ovarian suppression in women desiring fertility. The women who undergo surgery and are planned for ovarian stimulation or to undergo IVF are also not recommended to receive any ovarian suppression. Women who wish to delay treatment of infertility and who have undergone surgery for endometriosis may be given medical suppression to prevent recurrence of endometriosis, or in cases of residual disease where pregnancy is not planned. Women should be counseled to take suppressive therapy only till the pregnancy planning is begun. In a study, comparable pregnancy rates were found when suppression with letrozole, Gn-RH agonist was comapred with controls.[22]

There is no role of suppression of an ovary where the disease is severe as the reserve is already compromised and therefore no progesterone or estrogen plus progesterone or GnRH analog is suggested as it would further worsen the ovarian response to gonadotropins.

Role of Surgery in Advanced Endometriosis Prior to Ovarian Stimulation

There are specific indications in women with advanced endometriosis to undergo surgery prior to controlled ovarian stimulation and IVF. The recent ESHRE publication has changed the previous opinion and suggested that some women with advanced endometriosis may benefit from surgery and if the tubal status is considered good they can be considered for controlled ovarian stimulation alone with or without IVF. There are presently no data to recommend this; however, it is understood that these women are likely to need IVF. For optimizing the ovarian stimulation for ART, surgery becomes necessary as due to extensive disease, the ovarian cortex and stroma are not identified and there comes a role of careful drainage of the endometriosis with minimal removal of the cyst wall when the ovarian reserve is compromised, even if it is known that a complete removal of cyst wall should be attempted to prevent recurrence of disease. The presence of endometriomas can be a problem at the time of oocyte retrieval and in some cases may need surgery.

Oocyte Quality and Endometrioma

There is a pivotal role played by the oocyte where its genomics and metabolomics are at play to determine its embryonic competence. This has generally been studied indirectly by seeing the follicular fluid or the cumulus cells surrounding the oocyte.

Previous publications that were smaller had shown increased prevalence of morphological alterations of oocyte, such as the presence of dark central granulations, an abnormal zona pellucida, and/or other intra- and extra-cytoplasmic abnormalities.[24,25] Most of these publications were supportive of alteration in oocyte quality rather than a defect in endometrial receptivity in the context of endometriosis.[26]

The recent data have suggested that despite a decrease in the total number of mature oocytes retrieved and the number of embryos obtained, the rates of clinical pregnancy and delivery in IVF with or without intracytoplasmic sperm injection (ICSI) do not differ in patients with endometriosis compared with unaffected patients.[26-29]

OVARIAN STIMULATION IN IN VITRO FERTILIZATION IN WOMEN WITH ADVANCED ENDOMETRIOSIS

The aim of the ART cycle is to have controlled induced hyperstimulation in the ovary with all ovarian follicles developing equally till a trigger is given for retrieval of oocytes of appropriate stage and adequate numbers, which is often challenging in women with advanced disease and low ovarian reserve. The protocol for the optimal number of good follicles to be retrieved for the ART cycle needs to be individualized as per the parameters of the woman needing treatment. The most commonly used protocols are as follows.

Gonadotropin-releasing Hormone Agonist Protocol

This protocol is widely used and preferred in women with endometriosis as the risk of hyperstimulation is not likely in women especially with advanced disease. The initial use of GnRH agonist adds to a suppressive role and may have a theoretical benefit of suppressing the disease; however, the superiority of this protocol has not been validated in studies compared to antagonist-based ovarian stimulation cycles. In fact, the suppression caused by the daily use of GnRH agonist may have a suppressive effect and affect the number of follicles stimulated, thereby leading to cycle cancellation in women with poor response. This protocol can only be considered in women with normal range of AMH levels in women with endometriosis.

Long/Ultralong Gonadotropin-releasing Hormone Agonist Protocol

This protocol involved suppression of the pituitary by giving two to four GnRH long-acting depot injection for a period of 2–4 months causing hypoestrogenic state, thereby suppressing the endometriosis to lead to a low estrogenic state with theoretical advantage of improving the results of subsequent ovarian stimulation by human menopausal gonadotropins (hMG). There were multiple published studies to suggest improved pregnancy outcome with this protocol, and this became the protocol of choice. However, in advanced endometriosis where the reserve is compromised, this protocol produces marked suppression and therefore fewer follicles in women with low AMH. This may be used in women with deep infiltrating endometriosis where the AMH values are in normal range.

Gonadotropin-releasing Hormone Antagonist Cycle

The antagonist-based cycles are widely preferred as there is no suppression and all follicles are stimulated by a higher dose of gonadotropins from day 2 of cycle in the hope to attain plenty of follicles for retrieval. The recent ESHRE 2022 guideline does not suggest superiority of any protocol for ART.

Various trials have evaluated GnRH antagonist versus GnRH agonist ovarian stimulation protocols in women with endometriosis. An observational retrospective analysis as well as a randomized control trial (RCT) showed that the implantation and clinical pregnancy rates between the two protocols were comparable and none was inferior to the other.[30]

When the long GnRH agonist protocol was compared with the antagonist protocol, the studies did not show any significant difference in the outcome, especially with frozen embryo cycle; however, there was a nonsignificant better outcome in agonist cycles with agonist use.[31]

The other studies did find a favorable outcome when using a long GnRH agonist protocol in women who had stage I/II disease, but in women with III/IV disease, the antagonist was comparable or better than the long agonist suppressed cycles.[32]

Based on the above published data, the ESHRE suggested that no specific protocol for ART in women with endometriosis can be recommended. Either GnRH antagonist or agonist protocols can be offered based on patients' and physicians' preferences as no difference in pregnancy rates or live birth rates has been demonstrated.

Luteal Phase Stimulation Protocols

Repeat stimulation in the luteal phase can be considered in poor responder women who have advanced grades of endometriosis. This plan aims to allow embryo pooling and then opt for "frozen embryo" transfer. The basic protocol is the same as any poor responder patient. Here, after the ovum pick-up, repeat ovarian stimulation is started from the very next day with HMG plus letrozole, and follicle monitoring is started after 5–7 days. If follicles do not show dominance on day 12, then progesterone (10 mg medroxyprogesterone acetate) is added, and gonadotropins are continued till a dominant follicle of 18 mm is obtained. Subsequent second oocyte retrieval is carried out following 10,000 IU human chorionic gonadotropin (HCG) trigger.[33]

Luteal phase ovarian stimulation (LPOS) refers to the initiation of ovarian stimulation directly in the luteal phase. This is based on the concept of multiple follicular recruitment waves in a single menstrual cycle.[34] LPOS was initially designed for cancer patients needing fertility preservation.[35,36] It is now used in infertile women with poor response during the follicular phase.[37,38] In poor ovarian responders (PORs), LPOS may yield more competent oocytes and embryos, compared to follicular phase ovarian stimulation.[33,39,40] High levels of progesterone present physiologically during the luteal phase may block a premature luteinizing hormone (LH) surge, which is more frequent in PORs to ovarian stimulation during the follicular phase.

Double Stimulation in Poor Responders

In 2014, Kuang proposed "Shanghai Protocol," a new protocol. He used the LPOS following oocyte retrieval, in the same cycle when follicular phase ovarian stimulation had also been carried out. With the main aim of getting more oocytes in a short period of time, they used letrozole or clomiphene citrate plus HMG. They used GnRH antagonist to suppress ovarian LH surge and its triggering with GnRH agonist, along with total embryo vitrification. This was followed by second stimulation, and therefore it was also called double ovarian stimulation.[41]

The double stimulation protocols can be used in women who are poor responders with endometriosis where the first stimulation (follicular phase stimulation) fails to yield an adequate number of oocytes. The repeat stimulation is carried out in the luteal phase. In the first phase, the trigger used is GnRH agonist; subsequent to oocyte retrieval, the second phase stimulation is begun. This differs from luteal phase stimulation where the stimulation is started in the luteal phase where there is no or minimal stimulation attempted in the follicular phase. The second-phase stimulation protocol is actually same as luteal phase stimulation described above.

Progesterone Primed Ovarian Stimulation Protocol for Women with Endometriosis

Progesterone primed ovarian stimulation (PPOS) is a newer protocol where the progesterone supplementation is given in the beginning of the ovarian stimulation. The PPOS protocol causes pituitary suppression by oral progestins, started along with the gonadotropins. Recent publication in 2020 has showed that the PPOS protocol could be a choice for women with endometriosis undergoing fertility preservation.[42]

The PPOS protocol could be more advantageous in planned "freeze-all" cycles, such as oocyte donation, preimplantation genetic testing (PGT), and fertility preservation. However, till more experience is gained, the evidence is limited to support this protocol, but it does seem promising.[43-45]

Using Donor Oocyte Versus Self-Oocyte

Initial data suggested the presence of endometrioma impacting the oocyte quality, but present data do not suggest that the oocytes are of inferior quality. Hence, there is no evidence to suggest these women to opt for donor eggs until the stimulation response is very poor, which in itself is an indication for donor oocytes.

LUTEAL PHASE SUPPORT FOR WOMEN WITH ADVANCED ENDOMETRIOSIS

There are studies that do suggest that the overall pregnancy rates are poorer when infertile women with endometriosis were compared to women with tubal fertility. However, when the bias was removed and the factors were confounded, it showed similar IVF outcomes. The role of which progestogen is chosen for luteal phase is not well defined; however, from personnel experience, I have preference for dydrogesterone molecule in women with endometriosis. There are few studies that do suggest the immunomodulatory effect of retroprogesterone and also its anti-inflammatory action, may be adding to the advantage of using this molecule for luteal support.[46]

CONCLUSION

COS in endometriosis may be affected by endometriosis itself, surgery done for endometriosis and age. Ovarian tissue damage induced by endometriosis is a result of inflammatory reaction and mechanical damage which affects the ovarian reserve and ovulation rate, ovarian response to controlled ovarian stimulation and pregnancy rates. Decreased AMH and altered ovarian follicle Cohort has been seen not only in patients with severe endometriosis but also in infertile patients with mild-to- minimal endometriosis.

There is a lower rate of spontaneous ovulation in unoperated ovaries with an endometrioma and a progressive decline in ovarian reserve with progressive reduction in AMH serum levels, which is faster than in healthy controls is observed. Surgery for endometrioma also reduces the ovarian reserve as low AMH and AFC seen post-surgery. Thus, a tailored therapy for endometrioma is necessary. If operated a meticulous technique should be used. It is questionable to operate on endometriomas before COS for ART.

Therefore clinicians are not recommended to routinely perform surgery for ovarian endometrioma prior to ART to improve LBRs, as the current evidence shows no benefit and surgery is likely to have a negative impact on ovarian reserve. Surgery for endometrioma prior to ART can be considered to improve endometriosis-associated pain or accessibility of follicles. COS in women with endometrioma is associated with lower response, higher dose of GT for stimulation, poor response lower number and quality of oocytes obtained. Ovarian responsiveness was significantly associated with the size and number of endometriomas and reduction in ovarian responsiveness could be observed only in presence of larger cysts (>5 cm) and in those with bilateral cysts. Initial dose should be determined by the patient's age, ovarian reserve (AFC and AMH), body mass index, and response to prior stimulation regime if available. Dose was then adjusted according to the response of ovarian follicles, which were followed-up via vaginal ultrasonography. There is no evidence of a preference for FSH or hMG, though LH activity gives better response in those with low ovarian reserve.

KEY MESSAGES

- Clinicians have to face the challenge of selection of GT starting dose.
- Inadequate starting dose leads to insufficient follicular recruitment, which results in iatrogenic poor ovarian response.
- On the contrary, excessive starting dose is associated with excessive recruitment of follicles, leading to an increased incidence of OHSS.
- Advised to assess ovarian reserve (AMH and AFC) prior to deciding the dose
- High starting dose may increase P4 level during COS, and finally increases the cancellation rate of transfer in fresh cycles or decreases the PRs due to unsynchronized development of endometrium.
- Implantation rate (IR), clinical pregnancy rate (CPR), ongoing pregnancy rate (OPR), live birth rate (LBR) and cumulative LBRs after COS in a GnRH antagonist cycle were not inferior to those for a GnRH agonist protocol
- The administration of GnRH agonist prior to ART treatment to improve LBR in infertile women with endometriosis is not recommended, as the benefit is uncertain. Very low-quality evidence.
- In all endometriosis groups, patients treated with the agonist protocol have a significantly higher number of MII oocytes and available embryos that can be cryopreserved compared to patients treated with the antagonist protocol.
- As surgery may affect the response to COS, one should identify patients that may benefit from ART after surgery.
- Endometriosis fertility index (EFI) should be used as it is validated, reproducible and cost-effective.

■ REFERENCES

1. Burney RO, Giudice LC. Pathogenesis and pathophysiology of endometriosis. Fertil Steril. 2012;98(3):511-9.
2. Practice Committee of the American Society for Reproductive Medicine. Endometriosis and infertility: a committee opinion. Fertil Steril. 2012;98:591-8.

3. Prescott J, Farland LV, Tobias DK, Gaskins AJ, Spiegelman D, Chavarro JE, et al. A prospective cohort study of endometriosis and subsequent risk of infertility. Hum Reprod. 2016;31:1475-82.
4. Da Broi MG, Ferriani RA, Navarro PA. Etiopathogenic mechanisms of endometriosis-related infertility. JBRA Assist Reprod. 2019;23(3):273-80.
5. American Society for Reproductive Medicine. Revised American Society for Reproductive Medicine classification of endometriosis: 1996. Fertil Steril. 1997;67(5):817-21.
6. Adamson GD, Pasta DJ. Endometriosis fertility index: the new, validated endometriosis staging system. Fertil Steril. 2010;94:1609-15.
7. Tomassetti C, Geysenbergh B, Meuleman C, Timmerman D, Fieuws S, D'Hooghe T. External validation of the endometriosis fertility index (EFI) staging system for predicting non-ART pregnancy after endometriosis surgery. Hum Reprod. 2013;28:1280-8.
8. Boujenah J, Bonneau C, Hugues JN, Sifer C, Poncelet C. External validation of the endometriosis fertility index in a French population. Fertil Steril. 2015;104:119-23.e1.
9. Raffi F, Metwally M, Amer S. The impact of excision of ovarian endometrioma on ovarian reserve: a systematic review and meta-analysis. J Clin Endocrinol Metab. 2012;97:3146-54.
10. Somigliana E, Berlanda N, Benaglia L, Viganò P, Vercellini P, Fedele L. Surgical excision of endometriomas and ovarian reserve: a systematic review on serum antimüllerian hormone level modifications. Fertil Steril. 2012;98:1531-8.
11. Wang Y, Ruan X, Lu D, Sheng J, Mueck AO. Effect of laparoscopic endometrioma cystectomy on anti-Müllerian hormone (AMH) levels. Gynecol Endocrinol. 2019;35(6):494-7.
12. Muzii L, Di Tucci C, Di Feliciantonio M, Galati G, Di Donato V, Musella A, et al. Antimüllerian hormone is reduced in the presence of ovarian endometriomas: a systematic review and meta-analysis. Fertil Steril. 2018;110(5):932-40.e1.
13. Uncu G, Kasapoglu I, Ozerkan K, Seyhan A, Yilmaztepe AO, Ata B. Prospective assessment of the impact of endometriomas and their removal on ovarian reserve and determinants of the rate of decline in ovarian reserve. Hum Reprod. 2013;28(8):2140-5.
14. Yoo JH, Cha SH, Park CW, Kim JY, Yang KM, Song IO, et al. Serum anti-Müllerian hormone is a better predictor of ovarian response than FSH and age in IVF patients with endometriosis. Clin Exp Reprod Med. 2011;38(4):222-7.
15. Falconer H, Sundqvist J, Gemzell-Danielsson K, von Schoultz B, D'Hooghe TM, Fried G. IVF outcome in women with endometriosis in relation to tumour necrosis factor and anti-Müllerian hormone. Reprod Biomed Online. 2009;18(4):582-8.
16. Marcellin L, Santulli P, Bourdon M, Comte C, Maignien C, Just PA, et al. Serum antimüllerian hormone concentration increases with ovarian endometrioma size. Fertil Steril. 2019;111(5):5944-52.
17. Roman H, Chanavaz-Lacheray I, Mircea O, Berby B, Dehan L, Braund S, et al. Large ovarian endometriomas associated with high preoperative anti-Müllerian hormone levels. RBM Online. 2021;42(1):158-64.
18. McLaren J, Prentice A, Charnock-Jones DS, Smith SK. Vascular endothelial growth factor (VEGF) concentrations are elevated in peritoneal fluid of women with endometriosis. Hum Reprod. 1996;11:220-3.

19. Bourlev V, Volkov N, Pavlovitch S, Lets N, Larsson A, Olovsson M. The relationship between micro-vessel density, proliferative activity and expression of vascular endothelial growth factor-A and its receptors in eutopic endometrium and endometriotic lesions. Reproduction. 2006;132:501-9.
20. Becker CM, Bokor A, Heikinheimo O, Horne A, Jansen F, Kiesel L, et al. ESHRE Endometriosis Guideline Group, ESHRE guideline: endometriosis. Hum Reprod Open. 2022;2:2022.
21. Hughes E, Brown J, Collins JJ, Farquhar C, Fedorkow DM, Vanderkerchove P. Ovulation suppression for endometriosis for women with subfertility. Cochrane Database Syst Rev. 2007;2007(3):CD000155.
22. Alborzi S, Hamedi B, Omidvar A, Dehbashi S, Alborzi S, Alborzi M. A comparison of the effect of short-term aromatase inhibitor (letrozole) and GnRH agonist (triptorelin) versus case control on pregnancy rate and symptom and sign recurrence after laparoscopic treatment of endometriosis. Arch Gynecol Obstet. 2011;284:105-10.
23. Benschop L, Farquhar C, van der Poel N, Heineman MJ. Interventions for women with endometrioma prior to assisted reproductive technology. Cochrane Database Syst Rev. 2010;(11):CD008571.
24. Ceviren A, Urfan A, Donmez L, Isikoglu M. Characteristic cytoplasmic morphology of oocytes in endometriosis patients and its effect on the outcome of assisted reproduction treatments cycles. IVF Lite. 2014;1:88-93.
25. Goud PT, Goud AP, Joshi N, Puscheck E, Diamond MP, Abu-Soud HM. Dynamics of nitric oxide, altered follicular microenvironment, and oocyte quality in women with endometriosis. Fertil Steril. 2014;102(1):151-9.e5.
26. Sharma S, Roy Choudhury S, Bathwal S, Bhattacharya R, Kalapahar S, Chattopadhyay R, et al. Pregnancy and live birth rates are comparable in young infertile women presenting with severe endometriosis and tubal infertility. Reprod Sci. 2020;27(6):1340-9.
27. Gonzalez-Comadran M, Schwarze JE, Zegers-Hochschild F, Souza MD, Carreras R, Checa MA. The impact of endometriosis on the outcome of assisted reproductive technology. Reprod Biol Endocrinol. 2017;15(1):8.
28. Murta M, Machado RC, Zegers-Hochschild F, Checa MA, Sampaio M, Geber S. Endometriosis does not affect live birth rates of patients submitted to assisted reproduction techniques: analysis of the Latin American Network Registry database from 1995 to 2011. J Assist Reprod Genet. 2018;35(8):1395-9.
29. Yang C, Geng Y, Li Y, Chen C, Gao Y. Impact of ovarian endometrioma on ovarian responsiveness and IVF: a systematic review and meta-analysis. Reprod Biomed Online. 2015;31(1):9-19.
30. Pabuccu R, Onalan G, Kaya C. GnRH agonist and antagonist protocols for stage I-II endometriosis and endometrioma in in vitro fertilization/intracytoplasmic sperm injection cycles. Fertil Steril. 2007;88:832-9.
31. Rodriguez-Purata J, Coroleu B, Tur R, Carrasco B, Rodriguez I, Barri PN. Endometriosis and IVF: are agonists really better? Analysis of 1180 cycles with the propensity score matching. Gynecol Endocrinol. 2013;29:859-62.
32. Drakopoulos P, Rosetti J, Pluchino N, Blockeel C, Santos-Ribeiro S, de Brucker M, et al. Does the type of GnRH analogue used, affect live birth rates in women with endometriosis undergoing IVF/ICSI treatment, according to the rAFS stage? Gynecol Endocrinol. 2018;34:884-9.

33. Wei LH, Ma WH, Tang N, Wei JH. Luteal-phase ovarian stimulation is a feasible method for poor ovarian responders undergoing in vitro fertilization/intracytoplasmic sperm injection-embryo transfer treatment compared to a GnRH antagonist protocol: a retrospective study. Taiwan J Obstet Gynecol. 2016;55:50-4.
34. Baerwald AR, Adams GP, Pierson RA. Ovarian antral folliculogenesis during the human menstrual cycle: a review. Hum Reprod Update. 2012;18:73-91.
35. Cakmak H, Katz A, Cedars MI, Rosen MP. Effective method for emergency fertility preservation: random-start controlled ovarian stimulation. Fertil Steril. 2013;100:1673-80.
36. von Wolff M, Thaler CJ, Frambach T, Zeeb C, Lawrenz B, Popovici RM, et al. Ovarian stimulation to cryopreserve fertilized oocytes in cancer patients can be started in the luteal phase. Fertil Steril. 2009;92:1360-5.
37. Martinez F, Clua E, Devesa M, Rodriguez I, Arroyo G, Gonzalez C, et al. Comparison of starting ovarian stimulation on day 2 versus day 15 of the menstrual cycle in the same oocyte donor and pregnancy rates among the corresponding recipients of vitrified oocytes. Fertil Steril. 2014;102:1307-11.
38. Qin N, Chen Q, Hong Q, Cai R, Gao H, Wang Y, et al. Flexibility in starting ovarian stimulation at different phases of the menstrual cycle for treatment of infertile women with the use of in vitro fertilization or intracytoplasmic sperm injection. Fertil Steril. 2016;106:334-41.e1.
39. Lin LT, Vitale SG, Chen SN, Wen ZH, Tsai HW, Chern CU, et al. Luteal phase ovarian stimulation may improve oocyte retrieval and oocyte quality in poor ovarian responders undergoing in vitro fertilization: preliminary results from a single-center prospective pilot study. Adv Ther. 2018;35:847-56.
40. Li Y, Yang W, Chen X, Li L, Zhang Q, Yang D. Comparison between follicular stimulation and luteal stimulation protocols with clomiphene and HMG in women with poor ovarian response. Gynecol Endocrinol. 2016;32:74-7.
41. Kuang Y, Chen Q, Hong Q, Lyu Q, Ai A, Fu Y, et al. Double stimulations during the follicular and luteal phases of poor responders in IVF/ICSI programmes (Shanghai protocol). Reprod Biomed Online. 2014;29:684-91.
42. Mathieu d'Argent E, Ferrier C, Zacharopoulou C, Ahdad-Yata N, Boudy AS, Cantalloube A, et al. Outcomes of fertility preservation in women with endometriosis: comparison of progestin-primed ovarian stimulation versus antagonist protocols. J Ovarian Res. 2020;13(1):18.
43. Giles J, Alama P, Gamiz P, Vidal C, Badia P, Pellicer A, et al. Medroxyprogesterone acetate is a useful alternative to a gonadotropin-releasing hormone antagonist in oocyte donation: a randomized, controlled trial. Fertil Steril. 2021;116(2):404-12.
44. La Marca A, Capuzzo M, Sacchi S, Imbrogno MG, Spinella F, Varricchio MT, et al. Comparison of euploidy rates of blastocysts in women treated with progestins or GnRH antagonist to prevent the luteinizing hormone surge during ovarian stimulation. Hum Reprod. 2020;35(6):1325-31.
45. Chen J, Cheng Y, Fu W, Peng X, Sun X, Chen H, et al. PPOS protocol effectively improves the IVF outcome without increasing the recurrence rate in early endometrioid endometrial cancer and atypical endometrial hyperplasia patients after fertility preserving treatment. Front Med. 2021;8:581927.
46. Chao P, Yan H, Yingfang Z. Dydrogesterone in the treatment of endometriosis: evidence mapping and meta-analysis. Arch Gynecol Obstet. 2021;304:231-52.

Chapter 8

Stages of Reproductive Aging and Correlation with Symptoms

Sarita Bhalerao, Priya Vora

■ INTRODUCTION

The menopause transition period is of clinical significance as it is marked by a number of changes in health and life quality as well as long-term changes in health outcomes. Stages of Reproductive Aging Workshop (STRAW) in 2001 proposed a nomenclature and a system to stage ovarian aging, which included menstrual and qualitative hormonal criteria to define each stage.

The STRAW staging system is regarded as the gold standard for characterizing reproductive aging through menopause. The criteria evaluated by STRAW participants were menstrual cycles, hormonal parameters including estradiol follicle-stimulating hormone (FSH), inhibin B, anti-Müllerian hormone (AMH), menopausal symptoms, fertility, and antral follicle count (AFC).

■ STRAW STAGING SYSTEM (2001)

STRAW Staging System (2001) divided an adult female life into *three* stages:
1. Reproductive
2. Menopausal transition
3. Postmenopause.

These three phases comprised a total of seven stages centered on the final menstrual period (FMP) (stage 0). The reproductive phase was divided into stages –5, –4, and –3, corresponding to early, peak, and late, respectively. The menopausal transition phase consisted of stages –2 (early) and –1 (late), and the postmenopause phase contained stages +1 (early) and +2 (late).[1,2]

The *reproductive phase* has been divided into early, peak, and late.

Late Reproductive Stage (Stage –3)

The late reproductive stage is marked by a decrease in fecundability and changes in the menstrual cycle. Crucial hormonal parameters begin to change prior to apparent changes in the menstrual cycle. Fertility might still be possible, but the chances are lesser than that in the previous years. There is a diminishing follicle pool and the ovarian reserve varies in this period. The menstrual cycles are regular, but there may be a slight increase in variability of menstrual cycle length. FSH values are normal to a variable. As the follicle cohort shrinks, less inhibin B is produced, which leads to a rise in FSH.[3]

The late reproductive stage is subdivided into two substages (-3b and -3a) as suggested by STRAW + 10 (**Tables 1 and 2**).

In stage-3b, the length of the menstrual cycle and regularity is maintained without change in early follicular phase FSH levels. In this phase, AMH, inhibin B, and AFC are low in most studies.

In stage-3a, shorter menstrual cycles specifically start. FSH increases in the early follicular phase and becomes more variable, with the other three markers of ovarian aging being low.

Early Menopausal Transition (Stage–2)

In this, the ovarian follicle cohort is highly diminished. There is a fluctuation in the menstrual cycle length which exceeds 7 days. Inhibin B, AMH, and AFC reduce drastically. FSH is elevated more often. This rising FSH causes rapid folliculogenesis and a shorter follicular phase of the menstrual cycle.[4] Follicular growth has been observed in the luteal phase, which contributes to the formation of the dominant follicle of the next cycle before the onset of menses.[5] This leads to the further menstrual irregularity of menopause transition. Lower luteal progesterone levels, higher FSH levels, and unpredictable estrogen secretory patterns are observed.[6]

Late Menopausal Transition (Stage –1)

Amenorrhea for 60 days or longer marks this stage. Periods become very scanty and irregular. The presence of longer periods of amenorrhea marks a *sharp increase in menopausal symptoms*. During this phase, FSH levels may be raised into the menopausal range. FSH levels >25 IU/L are observed. This stage usually lasts for 1–3 years. Vasomotor symptoms (VMS) are more pronounced and occur in this stage.

The early menopause transition stage is attained by 47 years of age, the late menopause transition stage at 49 years, and the FMP occurs at 51 years of age in the majority of women.

Early Postmenopause (Stages +1a, +1b, and +1c)

Follicle-stimulating hormone continues to increase and estradiol continues to decrease until 2 years after the FMP. The levels of each of these hormones stabilize eventually. Early postmenopause is subdivided into three stages (+1a, +1b, and +1c).

The first two stages, +1a and +1b, are each 1 year long and end with the stabilization of FSH and estradiol.[7]

TABLE 1: STRAW + 10 staging system.

Stage	-5	-4	-3B	-3A	-2	-1	+1A	+1B	+1C	+2
	Menarche →						FMP (0) →			
Terminology	Early	Peak	Late		Early	Late	Early		Late	
	Reproductive				Menopausal transition		Postmenopause			
					Perimenopause					
Duration	Variable				Variable	1–3 years	2 years (1 + 1)		3–6 years	Remaining life span
Principal criteria										
Menstrual cycle	Variable to regular	Regular	Regular	Subtle changes in flow length	Variable length persistent ≥7-day difference in length of consecutive cycles	Interval of amenorrhea of ≥60 days				
Supportive criteria										
Endocrine				Variable	↑Variable	↑>25 IU/L	↑Variable		Stabilizes	
FSH			Low	Low	Low	Low	Low		Very low	
AMH			Low	Low	Low	Low	Low		Very low	
Inhibin B										
Antral follicle count			Low	Low	Low	Low	Very low		Very low	
Descriptive characteristics										
Symptoms						Vasomotor symptoms likely	Vasomotor symptoms most likely			Increasing symptoms of urogenital atrophy

(AMH: anti-Müllerian hormone; FSH: follicle-stimulating hormone)

Source: Harlow SD, Gass M, Hall J, Sluss PM, de Villiers TJ, STRAW + 10 Collaborative Group. Executive summary of the Stages of Reproductive Aging Workshop + 10: addressing the unfinished agenda of staging reproductive aging. Fertil Steril. 2012;97(4):843-51.

TABLE 2: Guidelines on Menopause-Recommendations IMS 2019–2020. Modified Anklesaria's Indian Menopause Society (IMS) consensus group staging.

Stage I	*Stage IIA*	*Stage IIB*	*Stage III3*
• Roughly 2 years before menopause • Early (premenopausal symptoms) • IA vasomotor instability • IB • Early psychosomatic symptoms • Menstrual problems	• 1 year after last period • Atrophic changes • Genitourinary • Vasomotor • Weight gain • Osteopenia	• Up to 5 years after menopause intermediate (postmenopausal symptoms) • Late psychosomatic and genital symptoms • Sexual disorders • Residual changes from stage IIA • Osteopenia or osteoporosis	• From 5 years post menopause till late (postmenopausal) complications: – Residual changes from stage II – Ischemic heart changes – Other late complications, e.g., Alzheimer's disease, osteoporosis
• Prevent and treat	Treat	Treat	Treat and palliate

Source: Indian Menopause Society consensus statement (2008).

Rapid changes in mean FSH and estradiol levels are observed in stage +1b. During this stage, hot flashes and night sweats are likely to occur.

The third stage, which lasts for 3-6 years, is accompanied by the stabilization of high FSH levels and low estradiol values. The entire early postmenopause hence lasts approximately 5-8 years.

Late Post Menopause (Stage +2)

No major changes in the reproductive endocrine function during this period but somatic aging becomes a matter of concern. *Urogenital atrophy* and symptoms of *vaginal dryness* have become increasingly common.[8]

■ SYMPTOM CORRELATION

Vasomotor Symptoms

Vasomotor symptoms are an important feature that occur in many women during menopause. Recent studies indicated that 80% of premenopausal women suffer from hot flashes, which may be milder initially, progressively increasing from early to late menopausal transition.[9] Although it was earlier believed that estrogen withdrawal caused hot flashes, recent evidence has indicated that *elevated FSH* is an independent marker associated with VMS.

It has been observed that VMS are more prolonged in duration in women who presented with VMS in the perimenopausal period (11.8 years) as compared to those who presented with VMS in postmenopause (3.4 years).[10]

In the SWAN (Study of Women's Health Across the Nation) study, Japanese and Chinese women had overall shorter duration and lower rates of hot flashes than African-American women.[11] Women with high body mass index (BMI) experienced hot flashes for longer periods. Symptom severity was more during the menopausal transition but became milder after the FMP. Various studies have proven that smoking, depressed mood, and anxiety are associated with the increased occurrence of hot flashes. VMS are a risk factor for the development of cardiovascular diseases. One large study demonstrated that there was an increased risk of developing cardiovascular disease (CVD) in women with VMS.[12]

Vaginal and Sexual Symptoms

Vaginal and sexual symptoms are common in postmenopausal women, affecting one third to half of them.[13] However, some perimenopausal women may also experience these symptoms. Genitourinary syndrome of menopause is associated with thinning of the vaginal epithelium, a decrease in collagen and elastin content, and elevated vaginal pH due to declining estrogen.[14] Vaginal dryness causes a huge impact on sexual life. Earlier in the transition, there is increased pain during sexual intercourse, while later in the transition, there is a decrease in desire.

According to SWAN, 20 months before the FMP, there was a decline in sexual function, which was greatest in late transition and slowed down after menopause.[15]

Sleep and Mood Changes

Women in menopause transition experience disturbed sleep and mood changes. Vasomotor and psychological symptoms are linked with sleep disturbances. The incidence of insomnia is higher in women with more severe VMS.[16] Ohayon et al. demonstrated that the prevalence of hot flashes was 12.5% in premenopausal women, 79% in perimenopausal women, and 39.3% in postmenopausal women with insomnia rates of 36.5%, 56.6%, and 50.7%, respectively.[17] Melbourne Midlife Women's Health Project reported poor sleep patterns as women progressed through menopause, which stabilized postmenopause.[18] It was unclear whether the cause was estrogen withdrawal or other hormonal changes or simply related to aging.

Quality of life during the menopausal transition strongly impacts mood. The Center for Epidemiologic Studies Depression scale noted that the risk of adverse mood symptoms increased from 20 to 62% by early perimenopause as compared to premenopause.[19] The prevalence of psychological distress as reported by SWAN was 28.9% in the early menopausal transition, 25.6% in the late menopausal transition, and 22% in postmenopause.[20]

■ LIMITATIONS OF THE ORIGINAL STRAW

The staging system can be only applied to healthy women. It could not be applied to women who were smokers, women with a BMI >30 kg/m^2, and those who had undergone hysterectomy. Women who engaged in heavy aerobic exercise and women with chronic menstrual cycle irregularities, uterine abnormalities, or ovarian abnormalities or illnesses such as cancer were also excluded from this.

■ NEED FOR RESTAGING

Advances in research have expanded the knowledge of the crucial changes in hypothalamic–pituitary and ovarian functions that occur before and after the FMP.

The STRAW + 10 workshop achieved the following aims:
- To reevaluate criteria for the onset of late reproductive life and early menopausal transition, given new population-based data relating to FSH, AFC, AMH, and inhibin B
- To reevaluate criteria for staging postmenopause, given new population-based data on changes in FSH and estradiol concentrations after the FMP
- To reevaluate applicability to women based on variations in body size, lifestyle, characteristics, and health status
- To identify remaining gaps in scientific knowledge and research priorities. The cost of the tests should be taken into consideration especially in poor resopurce countries like India.

■ CONCLUSION

Perimenopause is marked by physiological changes. These changes influence a woman's quality of life and have important health concerns. The STRAW staging system is a standardized staging system for reproductive aging. This system can be used by clinicians to guide women for their health needs.

KEY MESSAGES
- STRAW + 10 simplified bleeding criteria for the early and late menopausal transition.
- STRAW + 10 provides a more comprehensive basis for assessing reproductive aging in research and clinical contexts.
- Application of the STRAW + 10 staging system should improve comparability of studies of midlife women and facilitate clinical decision making.
- One should consider menstrual cycle criteria to remain the most important criteria as there is lack of international standardization of biomarker assays. The cost and/or invasiveness of the biomarker assays might restrict its use in poor-resource countries.
- Biomarker criteria should be used as supportive criteria as there is lack of assay standardization.
- One should use criteria that are independent of age, symptoms, and pathology.
- Nonetheless, important knowledge gaps persist, and seven research priorities are identified.

■ REFERENCES

1. Soules MR, Sherman S, Parrott E, Rebar R, Santoro N, Utian W, et al. Executive summary: stages of reproductive aging workshop (STRAW). Climacteric. 2001;4:267-72.
2. Harlow SD, Gass M, Hall JE, Lobo R, Maki P, Rebar RW, et al. Executive summary of the stages of reproductive aging workshop + 10: addressing the unfinished agenda of staging reproductive aging. Menopause. 2012;19(4):387-95.
3. Santoro N. Perimenopause: from research to practice. Journal of Women's Health. 2016;25(4):332-9.
4. Santoro N, Isaac B, Neal-Perry G, Adel T, Weingart L, Nussbaum A, et al. Impaired folliculogenesis and ovulation in older reproductive aged women. J Clin Endocrinol Metab. 2003;88:5502-9.
5. Vanden Brink H, Chizen D, Hale G, Baerwald A. Age-related changes in major ovarian follicular wave dynamics during the human menstrual cycle. Menopause. 2013;20:1243-54.
6. Santoro N, Crawford SL, Lasley WL, Luborsky JL, Matthews KA, McConnell D, et al. Factors related to declining luteal function in women during the menopausal transition. J Clin Endocrinol Metab. 2008;93:1711-21.
7. Randolph Jr JF, Zheng H, Sowers MR, Crandall C, Crawford S, Gold EB, et al. Change in follicle-stimulating hormone and estradiol across the menopausal transition: effect of age at the final menstrual period. J Clin Endocrinol Metab. 2011;96:746-54.
8. Stiles M, Redmer J, Paddock E, Schrager S. Gynaecologic issues in geriatric women. J Womens Health (Larchmt). 2012;21:4-9.
9. Gallicchio L, Miller SR, Kiefer J, Greene T, Zacur HA, Flaws JA. Risk factors for hot flashes among women undergoing the menopausal transition: baseline results from the Midlife Women's Health Study. Menopause. 2015;22:1098-107.
10. Avis NE, Crawford SL, Greendale G, Bromberger JT, Everson-Rose SA, Gold EB, et al. Duration of menopausal vasomotor symptoms over the menopause transition. JAMA Intern Med. 2015;175:531-9.
11. Smith RL, Gallicchio L, Miller SR, Zacur HA, Flaws JA. Risk factors for extended duration and timing of peak severity of hot flashes. PLoS One. 2016;11:e0155079.
12. van den Berg MJ, Herber-Gast GC, van der Schouw YT. Is an unfavourable cardiovascular risk profile a risk factor for vasomotor menopausal symptoms? Results of a population-based cohort study. BJOG. 2015;122:1252-8.
13. Santoro N, Komi J. Prevalence and impact of vaginal symptoms among postmenopausal women. J Sex Med. 2009;6:2133-42.
14. Kim HK, Kang SY, Chung YJ, Kim JH, Kim MR. The recent review of the genitourinary syndrome of menopause. J Menopausal Med. 2015;21:65-71.
15. Avis NE, Colvin A, Karlamangla AS, Crawford S, Hess R, Waetjen LE, et al. Change in sexual functioning over the menopausal transition: results from the study of women's health across the nation. Menopause. 2017;24:379-90.
16. Kravitz HM, Joffe H. Sleep during the perimenopause: a SWAN story. Obstet Gynecol Clin North Am. 2011;38:567-86.
17. Ohayon MM. Severe hot flashes are associated with chronic insomnia. Arch Intern Med. 2006;166:1262-8.

18. Dennerstein L, Lehert P, Guthrie JR, Burger HG, Modeling women's health during the menopausal transition: a longitudinal analysis. Menopause. 2007;14:53-62.
19. Bromberger JT, Kravitz HM. Mood and menopause: findings from the Study of Women's Health Across the Nation (SWAN) over 10 years. Obstet Gynecol Clin North Am. 2011;38:609-25.
20. Cohen LS, Soares CN, Vitonis AF, Otto MW, Harlow BL. Risk for new onset of depression during the menopausal transition: the Harvard study of moods and cycles. Arch Gen Psychiatry. 2006;63:385-90.

Chapter 9

Prevention and Management of Ovarian Hyperstimulation Syndrome

Fessy Louis T, Meera Ravi Kumar

■ INTRODUCTION

Ovarian hyperstimulation syndrome (OHSS) is a preventable, iatrogenic, and multiorgan disorder associated with ovarian stimulation. Most cases are self-limiting, although occasionally life threatening. Moderate-to-severe OHSS occurs in approximately 1–5% of cycles.[1] The traditional description of the syndrome generally includes a spectrum of findings ranging from mild to severe and critical category. Severe OHSS can lead to serious complications, including pleural effusion, acute renal insufficiency, and venous thromboembolism.

■ PREVENTION OF OVARIAN HYPERSTIMULATION SYNDROME

- Total prevention of OHSS is still not possible. Identifying at-risk patients and individualizing treatment will reduce the incidence of OHSS considerably. It mainly involves the identification of patients at risk and prediction of development of OHSS, and in cases of OHSS, supportive therapy to prevent complications.
- *Risk factors for OHSS:*[2] There is fair evidence that young women (<35 years of age) with lower body mass index (BMI), polycystic ovary syndrome (PCOS), high-dose gonadotropin stimulation, gonadotropin-releasing hormone (GnRH) agonist protocol, human chorionic gonadotropin (hCG) for trigger or luteal support, previous OHSS, and multiple pregnancy are associated with an increased risk of OHSS. Antral follicle count (AFC) >24, elevated anti-Müllerian hormone (AMH) values (>3.4 ng/mL), peak estradiol (E2) levels (>3,500 pg/mL), development of ≥25 follicles, high number of oocytes retrieved (>24 oocytes) are risk factors for development of OHSS. These cutoff values need to be validated. (Grade B).
- *Prediction:* Ultrasound monitoring of ovarian stimulation response and E2 monitoring are the best predictors of high risk for developing OHSS.

Preventive Strategies

Metformin therapy for PCOS is a safe and effective insulin-sensitizing agent which reduces the risk of OHSS by inhibiting the secretion of vascular endothelial growth factor A (VEGF-A). Hyperandrogenism is reduced and the nonovulatory follicles are decreased and there is reduced estrogen. Recent meta-analysis[3] has shown that metformin reduces the risk of OHSS by 63%. A daily dose of 500–1,500 mg, 3–4 months prior to the ovarian stimulation, is recommended. The majority of the studies in the meta-analysis involved the use of metformin in GnRH agonist, and only one study used the GnRH antagonist protocol.[4]

Gonadotropin-releasing hormone antagonist protocol with agonist trigger: A recent Cochrane review[5] of 2016 showed that antagonist protocols are associated with a reduced risk of OHSS without a significant difference in the live birth rate when compared with agonist cycles (2.7 vs. 12%). GnRH antagonists will reduce the circulating E2 levels and the pituitary luteinizing hormone (LH) secretion. GnRH agonist trigger lasts for 24–36 hours which is sufficient for the oocyte maturation alone with no prolonged stimulation of corpora lutea.[6] Expression of genes related to steroidogenesis is less at the time of oocyte retrieval with reduced VEGF and inhibin B.[7] The hCG trigger where the half-life is 28 hours continues to stimulate the corpora lutea for the next 14 days. With antagonist protocol, GnRH agonist trigger can be given instead of hCG trigger to further reduce the chance of OHSS to <0.2%.[8] But we cannot do fresh embryo transfer with agonist trigger as endometrial receptivity will be reduced, and we will have to freeze all and transfer at a later date. There is good evidence for a GnRH antagonist protocol with GnRH agonist trigger[2] (Grade A). Other options for triggering final oocyte maturation would be recombinant LH which resembles a natural LH surge. However, due to the poor cost–benefit ratio, its use is limited in clinical practice as a trigger.

Individualized controlled ovarian stimulation (iCOS) and AMH-based follicle-stimulating hormone (FSH) dosing algorithm: iCOS protocols adjusting the dose and duration of gonadotropins for at-risk patients and a new concept of AMH algorithm can be used to select the starting dose of FSH, which allows appropriate stimulation with a low risk of OHSS.[9] There seemed to be an association between the number of oocytes retrieved and the occurrence of OHSS. The rationale for the study was to use a dose of gonadotropin that maintains a balance between safety and efficacy. Hence for patients with AMH value >2.5 ng/dL with a starting dose of 112 IU/day of highly purified human menopausal gonadotrophin (HP-HMG), which results in a limited number of oocytes without compromising the pregnancy rate, the risk of OHSS is low; however, this dose can be increased unless cancellation of fresh transfer is adopted for 10–15 oocytes.[10]

Avoiding adjunct GnRH agonist utilization: GnRH agonist will cause more gonadotropin dosage to be used. The late luteal phase FSH rise does not occur as a result of which there are more number of larger follicles, and even the smaller follicles do not become atretic. The use of GnRH agonist triggering is not possible in the agonist protocol, and the cost of stimulation will be more.

Avoidance of hCG for luteal phase support: Progesterone, when used instead of hCG, has shown to halve the risk of OHSS.[11,12]

Aspirin: The VEGF-A levels cause platelet activation and release of histamine, serotonin, platelet-derived growth factors, and lysophosphatidic acid that potentiates the physiology of OHSS. A total of 100 mg of aspirin with steroids starting from the day of stimulation uptill confirmation of pregnancy or menstrual bleeding reduced the incidence of severe OHSS[13] (Grade B).

Glucocorticoids and their synthetic derivatives in doses of 10 or 30 mg can act on the vascular smooth muscle to help in reducing the vascular permeability, decrease inflammatory response, and prevent edema formation. However, there is insufficient evidence to recommend the use of glucocorticoids for the prevention of OHSS.

Coasting: It is a strategy where the administration of gonadotropins is withheld along with hCG for a few days until the levels of serum estrogen have declined to acceptable levels. The duration of delay is usually 3-4 days without affecting oocyte quality, while cycle cancellation should be considered when the controlled drift period is >4 days. A Cochrane review[14] has shown no evidence of benefit in the use of coasting to prevent OHSS (Grade C).

Freezing of embryos: Freezing of all embryos and transferring them in a subsequent cycle reduce the risk of OHSS considerably. There was no difference in the cumulative ongoing pregnancy rate or live birth rate between the fresh and frozen embryo transfer and a significant reduction in the incidence of moderate or severe OHSS in frozen embryo transfer cycles.[15,16] This will not reduce the incidence of early onset OHSS but will reduce late-onset OHSS[17] (Grade B Evidence).

Cycle cancellation: A guaranteed method of eliminating OHSS is cycle cancellation and the withholding of hCG administration. There is an associated financial and emotional burden for the patient with this preventive strategy. ≥18 follicles of ≥11 mm during oxidative stress (OS) with GnRH antagonist protocol and >30 follicles of 12 mm during OS with long GnRH agonist protocol[18] predicted severe OHSS with 83% sensitivity rate with a specificity as high as 84%.[19] In GnRH agonist cycles with an ovarian response of ≥18 follicles, there is an increased risk of OHSS and preventative measures are recommended, which could include cycle cancellation.[4]

Dopamine agonists: These act on D2 receptors by causing endocytosis of VEGF receptor 2 and preventing the increase in vascular permeability. Cabergoline significantly reduces the follicular fluid mediators such as hepatocyte growth factor, insulin-like growth factor, inhibin B, and AMH. VEGF expression on human granulosa cells starts before the administration of hCG. Cabergoline 0.5 mg is taken daily from the day of hCG injection and is continued for 10 days. There is a moderate amount of evidence to show that dopamine agonists reduce the incidence but not the severity of OHSS, with similar pregnancy rate with routine use[20] (Grade A). Cabergoline has been started when the follicle size reaches 15 mm (which will be approximately 2 days before trigger) and is continued for 8 days and hence ending before the blastocyst transfer. The incidence of severe OHSS is 0.9%, moderate OHSS 9.5%, and no critical OHSS.[21]

Aromatase inhibitors: They inhibit the rate-limiting step in E2 production and help to reduce the excess E2 and OHSS risk; however, further studies are required before their use in the prevention of OHSS.

Albumin and hydroxyethyl starch (HES): There is a reduced incidence of OHSS by administration of 25% albumin at the time of oocyte retrieval. The mechanism of action is by binding to, and deactivating, vasoactive mediators, which increases the plasma oncotic pressure and counteracts the effects of angiotensin II. However, in the Cochrane review, only limited evidence of benefit (Grade C) was found which suggested a significant decrease in the incidence of severe OHSS. Further research is needed before its routine use. The routine use is not recommended.[22]

Calcium gluconate: This lowers the OHSS risk as evidenced by studies. Calcium gluconate reduces the cyclic adenosine monophosphate (cAMP)-dependent renin–angiotensin II activity, thereby reducing VEGF. Studies have shown that intravenous (IV) calcium infusion (10 mL of 10% calcium gluconate in 200 mL normal saline) on the day of oocyte retrieval and on days 1–3 after oocyte retrieval can decrease OHSS risk.[23]

In vitro maturation (IVM): Retrieval of immature oocytes is a safe alternative, but not as popular as the normal in vitro fertilization (IVF) as the pregnancy and implantation rates are low. With advancements in cryopreservation techniques, there has been an improvement in the clinical outcomes.[24]

IV fluid and electrolyte imbalance management: To prevent progression into severe and moderate OHSS, IV fluid management is required. By strict monitoring of electrolytes and hematocrit values and correcting the deficit reduce the progression and complications of OHSS. The use of colloids alone for the treatment of OHSS is not supported by sufficient evidence (Grade C).

Other Experimental Methods

Kisspeptin trigger: Kisspeptin-54 is used as a trigger for the release of GnRH pulse and thereby the release of FSH and LH.

VEGF antagonists: Vasopressin V1a receptor antagonist: Blocks vasopressin-induced VEGF secretion.

■ MANAGEMENT

It requires early recognition and prompt treatment. A detailed history of how the stimulation went should not be forgotten:
- What dose of gonadotropin was given?
- How many days?
- What protocol was used?
- How many follicles?
- How many eggs were retrieved?
- What was the trigger injection?
- Whether a fresh transfer was done?
- How many embryos were transferred?
- Whether the diagnosis of a PCOS was present?

Once the detailed history of the treatment is taken, symptoms of abdominal bloating, abdominal discomfort/pain for which any analgesics they might require, nausea and vomiting, breathlessness, reduced urine output, swelling, and associated comorbidities such as thrombosis should be looked for. Thrombosis in OHSS is seen in the upper body sites and involves the arterial system. There is need to probe on dizziness, loss of vision, and neck pain.

Examination

- *General:* Assess for dehydration, edema (pedal, vulval, and sacral), vitals recording, measure abdominal girth, and body weight.
- *Per abdomen:* Look for ascites, any palpable mass, signs of peritonism.
- *Respiratory system:* Assess for pleural effusion, pneumonia, pulmonary edema.

Investigations

Investigations include full blood count, hematocrit (hemoconcentration), C-reactive protein (severity), urea and electrolytes (hyponatremia and hyperkalemia), serum osmolality (hypoosmolality), liver function tests (elevated enzymes and reduced albumin), coagulation profile (elevated fibrinogen and reduced antithrombin), hCG (to determine the outcome of treatment cycle) if appropriate, and ultrasound scan to check for ovarian size and pelvic and abdominal free fluid. Consider ovarian Doppler if torsion is suspected.

Other tests that may be indicated include arterial blood gases, D-dimers, electrocardiogram (ECG)/echocardiogram, chest X-ray, computerized tomography pulmonary angiogram (CTPA), or ventilation/perfusion (V/Q) scan.

Differential Diagnosis

Differential diagnosis includes pelvic infection, pelvic abscess, appendicitis, ovarian torsion or cyst rupture, bowel perforation,[25] and ectopic pregnancy.

Outpatient Management

In mild–moderate OHSS and in selected cases of severe OHSS:
- Counseling about the intake–output monitoring is to be given.
- Antiemetics and analgesics should be given.
- It is better to avoid nonsteroidal anti-inflammatory drugs due to renal compromise.
- Paracetamol and codeine can be offered for the pain.
- Women with severe OHSS being managed on an outpatient basis should receive thromboprophylaxis with low molecular weight heparin (LMWH).
- Paracentesis of ascitic fluid may be carried out on an outpatient basis by the abdominal or the transvaginal route under ultrasound guidance.
- Investigations need to be repeated if symptoms and signs of worsening; otherwise, every 2–3 days, there should be an outpatient review.

Signs of Worsening

Signs of worsening indicate increasing abdominal distension and pain, shortness of breath, tachycardia or hypotension, reduced urine output (<1,000 mL/24 h) or positive fluid balance (>1,000 mL/24 h), Weight gain and increased abdominal girth, and increasing hematocrit (>45).

Inpatient Management

Indications for inpatient treatment being worsening of signs and symptoms, e.g., unable to take orally due to nausea and severe pain and unable to come for regular follow-up. Once the patient is admitted, the need for multidisciplinary team involvement is required in case of severe and critical OHSS. In critical OHSS, the patient needs to be managed in the intensive care unit (ICU). Daily monitoring of abdominal girth, body weight, intake–output, and blood investigations, such as hematocrit, serum electrolytes, osmolality, and liver function tests. Recovery is identified by diuresis reduction in hemoconcentration, reduced abdominal girth, and weight.[26,27] Abdominal girth and weight along with C-reactive protein are markers used for monitoring.[28]

Fluid Management

- Intake of oral fluids which is ideally guided by thirst but in cases of acute dehydration, crystalloids can be the first choice.
- 1–2 L of fluid is advised to be taken orally.
- When there is persistent hemoconcentration despite the above measure, colloid infusion with IV monitoring and anesthetic input has to be opted for.
- The multidisciplinary team needs to be involved if oliguria is not responding to paracentesis and volume replacement. This is the only instance where diuretics have a role in the management of oliguria.
- IV fluid infusion needs to be done with caution as there can be worsening of ascites.
- Colloid in the form of human albumin 25% is used may be used as a plasma volume expander in doses of 50–100 g, infused over 4 hours, and repeated every 4- to 12-hourly.[22,26]
- Strict fluid balance recording should be followed for these patients.[29]

Paracentesis

Paracentesis can be done by ultrasound guided either transvaginally or transabdominally. The procedure essentially reduced the intra-abdominal pressure, hence increasing the organ perfusion. It is done as a treatment for severe OHSS and has shown to reduce the duration of hospital stay. Thoracentesis is considered after careful assessment of the degree of respiratory compromise (Grade B). The indications for the procedure are severe symptoms, e.g., abdominal distension and abdominal pain, shortness of breath and respiratory compromise, and oliguria despite adequate volume replacement. The mean volume of fluid to be removed is 500–4,500 mL. But young patients tolerate more volumes of fluid removal at a time when compared to their older counterparts.[26,30] Autotransfusion can be done, thereby avoiding the potential allergic reaction involved with exogenous albumin infusion.

Thromboprophylaxis

In severe OHSS, there is always an increased risk of thromboembolism,[31] Especially when there is reduced mobility, obesity, and a preexisting thrombophilia. Severe OHSS per se increases the risk as there is vascular endothelial dysfunction and prothrombotic state due to the hemoconcentration.[32] As a prophylactic measure, mobilization, avoidance of dehydration, use of full-length graduated compressing stockings, and administration of LMWH can be done. For patients confined to bed, we can use intermittent pneumatic compression devices and where chemical thromboprophylaxis is contraindicated[33] once conceived, they need to continue it till the end of the first trimester.[33] Unusual neurological symptoms, even if they present several weeks after apparent improvement in OHSS, should not be taken lightly, and thromboembolism needs to be considered. The incidence is between 0.7 and 10%.

Surgical Management

Surgical management is required for adnexal torsion, ovarian rupture, or ectopic pregnancy. Hyperstimulated ovaries are highly vascular and liable to damage on handling; hence, surgery is to be performed by an experienced surgeon. At times, termination of pregnancy has been reported to be done for progressive thrombosis despite anticoagulation.

OVARIAN HYPERSTIMULATION SYNDROME AND PREGNANCY

There is an increased incidence of preeclampsia (21.2%) and prematurity (36%) in pregnancies complicated by OHSS.

CONCLUSION

Ovarian hyperstimulation syndrome can result in significant morbidity and even life-threatening complications in severe forms. With proper identification of patients at risk and monitoring the patients, we can decrease the incidence and progress of severity of OHSS effectively with available preventive strategies.

KEY MESSAGES

- Serious, detrimental, and unintended consequence of COS due to:
  - Excessive ovarian stimulation
  - Excessive ovarian response to COS
  - hCG used for triggering ovulation
- OHSS can be early because of stimulation or late when there is occurrence of pregnancy.
- Late OHSS is more likely to be severe than early OHSS.
- OHSS can be prevented by:
  - Identify high-risk patients and cycle
  - Use low-risk treatment
  - Specific measures in individual cases
- All women undergoing COS should be considered potentially at risk of developing OHSS.

Contd...

Prevention and Management of Ovarian Hyperstimulation Syndrome

Contd…

- Incidence of mild-to-moderate OHSS is 0.6–14% and that for severe is severe OHSS is 0.2–0.5% of 'conventional' IVF cycles
- Risk factors include:
  - PCOS
  - Excessive ovarian response
  - Younger women <30 years
  - Low BMI
  - High GT dose for OI
  - Increased hCG exposure—LPS with hCG and MP
  - Previous OHSS
- Key to prevention of OHSS is:
  - Experience with OI therapy and recognition of risk factors for OHSS
  - Highly individualized OI regimens carefully monitored with USG and E2
  - Use of minimum dose and duration of GT therapy necessary to achieve the therapeutic goal
- Prevention of OHSS can be implemented before stating stimulation, during stimulation and after ovulation or oocyte retrieval.
  - *Before:*
    - Identification of risk factors to individualize COS
    - Correct adaptation of stimulation protocols
    - Limit the dose or concentration of hCG
    - Monitoring COS using USG and E2 assays constitutes the 'gold standard'
    - Use of GnRH antagonist
    - Cycle cancellation or coasting
  - *During:*
    - Limit the dose or concentration of hCG
    - Use Rec LH/GnRH agonist to trigger ovulation
    - IVM
    - Prophylactic albumin in high risk
    - Transfer of single embryo MP rate thus OHSS
  - *After:*
    - Cryopreservation of all embryos for transfer in subsequent cycle
    - Using progesterone instead of hCG for luteal phase support
    - Dopamine agonist
    - Use of antagonist post-cryofreezing all embryos or with Fresh ET?
- GnRH antagonist protocol coupled with GnRHa triggering safe, simple and efficient methos of preventing OHSS.
- However, GnRH agonist trigger leads to lower luteal phase steroidal concentrations.
- LP and early pregnancy support with adequate E2 and P4 supplementation is essential for optimal outcome.
- Single blastocyst transfer is strongly recommended.
- LPS with low doses of hCG in high-risk patients, secure a normal pregnancy outcome.
- A significantly higher rate of early pregnancy loss in the GnRHa group.
- Freeze all with FET is the best option with good PRS.

■ REFERENCES

1. Steward RG, Lan L, Shah AA, Yeh JS, Price TM, Goldfarb JM, et al. Oocyte number as a predictor for ovarian hyperstimulation syndrome and live birth: an analysis of 256,381 in vitro fertilization cycles. Fertil Steril. 2014;101:967-73.
2. Practice Committee of the American Society for Reproductive Medicine. Prevention and treatment of moderate and severe ovarian hyperstimulation syndrome: a guideline. Fertil Steril. 2016;106(7):1634-47.
3. Huang X, Wang P, Tal R, Lv F, Li Y, Zhang X. A systematic review and meta-analysis of metformin among patients with polycystic ovary syndrome undergoing assisted reproductive technology procedures. Int J Gynaecol Obstet. 2015;131:111-6.
4. ESHRE Guideline Group on Ovarian Stimulation, Bosch E, Broer S, Griesinger G, Grynberg M, Humaidan P, Kolibianakis E, Kunicki M, La Marca A, Lainas G, Le Clef N. ESHRE guideline: ovarian stimulation for IVF/ICSI. Human Reproduction Open. 2020;2020(2).
5. Al-Inany HG, Youssef MA, Aboulghar M, Broekmans F, Sterrenburg M, Smit J, et al. Gonadotrophin-releasing hormone antagonists for assisted reproductive technology. Cochrane Database Syst Rev. 2011;(5):CD001750.
6. Griesinger G, Diedrich K, Devroey P, Kolibianakis EM. GnRH agonist for triggering final oocyte maturation in the GnRH antagonist ovarian hyperstimulation protocol: a systematic review and meta-analysis. Hum Reprod Update. 2006;12(2):159-68.
7. Haas J, Ophir L, Barzilay E, Yerushalmi GM, Yung Y, Kedem A, et al. GnRH agonist vs. hCG for triggering of ovulation—differential effects on gene expression in human granulosa cells. PLoS One. 2014;9(3):e90359.
8. Youssef MAFM, Van der Veen F, Al-Inany HG, Mochtar MH, Griesinger G, Nagi Mohesen M, et al. Gonadotropin-releasing hormone agonist versus hCG for oocyte triggering in antagonist-assisted reproductive technology. Cochrane Database Syst Rev. 2014;(10):CD008046.
9. Sopa N, Larsen EC, Westring Hvidman H, Andersen AN. An AMH-based FSH dosing algorithm for OHSS risk reduction in first cycle antagonist protocol for IVF/ICSI. Eur J Obstet Gynecol Reprod Biol. 2019;237:42-7.
10. Magnusson Å, Källen K, Thurin-Kjellberg A, Bergh C. The number of oocytes retrieved during IVF: a balance between efficacy and safety. Hum Reprod. 2018;33(1):58-64.
11. van der Linden M, Buckingham K, Farquhar C, Kremer JAM, Metwally M. Luteal phase support for assisted reproduction cycles. Cochrane Database Syst Rev. 2015;2015(7):CD009154.
12. Humaidan P, Polyzos NP, Alsbjerg B, Erb K, Mikkelsen AL, Elbaek HO, et al. GnRHa trigger and individualized luteal phase hCG support according to ovarian response to stimulation: two prospective randomized controlled multi-centre studies in IVF patients. Hum Reprod. 2013;28(9):2511-21.
13. Revelli A, Dolfin E, Gennarelli G, Lantieri T, Massobrio M, Holte JG, et al. Low-dose acetylsalicylic acid plus prednisolone as an adjuvant treatment in IVF: a prospective, randomized study. Fertil Steril. 2008;90(5):1685-91.
14. D'Angelo A, Brown J, Amso NN. Coasting (withholding gonadotrophins) for preventing ovarian hyperstimulation syndrome. Cochrane Database Syst Rev. 2011;(2):CD002811.

15. Vuong LN, Dang VQ, Ho TM, Huynh BG, Ha DT, Pham TD, et al. IVF transfer of fresh or frozen embryos in women without polycystic ovaries. N Engl J Med. 2018;378:137-47.
16. Shi Y, Sun Y, Hao C, Zhang H, Wei D, Zhang Y, et al. Transfer of fresh versus frozen embryos in ovulatory women. N Engl J Med. 2018;378:126-36.
17. D'Angelo A, Amso N. Embryo freezing for preventing ovarian hyperstimulation syndrome. Cochrane Database Syst Rev. 2007;(3):CD002806.
18. Mathur RS, Akande AV, Keay SD, Hunt LP, Jenkins JM. Distinction between early and late ovarian hyperstimulation syndrome. Fertil Steril. 2000;73:901-7.
19. Papanikolaou EG, Pozzobon C, Kolibianakis EM, Camus M, Tournaye H, Fatemi HM, et al. Incidence and prediction of ovarian hyperstimulation syndrome in women undergoing gonadotropin-releasing hormone antagonist in vitro fertilization cycles. Fertil Steril. 2006;85:112-20.
20. Tang H, Mourad S, Zhai SD, Hart RJ. Dopamine agonists for preventing ovarian hyperstimulation syndrome. Cochrane Database Syst Rev. 2016;11(11):CD008605.
21. Gaafar S, El-Gezary D, El Maghraby HA. Early onset of cabergoline therapy for prophylaxis from ovarian hyperstimulation syndrome (OHSS): a potentially safer and more effective protocol. Reprod Biol. 2019;19(2):145-8.
22. Youssef MA, Mourad S. Volume expanders for the prevention of ovarian hyperstimulation syndrome. Cochrane Database Syst Rev. 2016;2016(8):CD001302.
23. Naredi N, Karunakaran S. Calcium gluconate infusion is as effective as the vascular endothelial growth factor antagonist cabergoline for the prevention of ovarian hyperstimulation syndrome. J Hum Reprod Sci. 2013;6:248.
24. Huang JY, Chian RC, Tan SL. Ovarian hyperstimulation syndrome prevention strategies: in vitro maturation. Semin Reprod Med. 2010;28(6):519-31.
25. Memarzadeh MT. A fatal case of ovarian hyperstimulation syndrome with perforated duodenal ulcer. Hum Reprod. 2010;25:808-9.
26. Practice Committee of the American Society for Reproductive Medicine. Ovarian hyperstimulation syndrome. Fertil Steril. 2008;90(Suppl. 5):S188-93.
27. Fábregues F, Balasch J, Manau D, Jiménez W, Arroyo V, Creus M, et al. Haematocrit, leukocyte and platelet counts and the severity of the ovarian hyperstimulation syndrome. Hum Reprod. 1998;13:2406-10.
28. Nowicka MA, Fritz-Rdzanek A, Grzybowski W, Walecka I, Niemiec KT, Jakimiuk AJ. C-reactive protein as the indicator of severity in ovarian hyperstimulation syndrome. Gynecol Endocrinol. 2010;26:399-403.
29. Delvigne A, Rozenberg S. Review of clinical course and treatment of ovarian hyperstimulation syndrome (OHSS). Hum Reprod Update. 2003;9:77-96.
30. Royal College of Obstetricians and Gynaecologists. Management of ascites in ovarian cancer patients (Scientific Impact Paper No. 45). RCOG. 2014.
31. Wormer KC, Jangda AA, El Sayed FA, Stewart KI, Mumford SL, Segars JH. Is thromboprophylaxis cost effective in ovarian hyperstimulation syndrome: a systematic review and cost analysis. Eur J Obstet Gynecol Reprod Biol. 2018;224:117-24.
32. Royal College of Obstetricians and Gynaecologists. Reducing the risk of venous thromboembolism during pregnancy and the puerperium (Green-top Guideline No. 37a). RCOG. 2015.
33. ESHRE Capri Workshop Group. Venous thromboembolism in women: a specific reproductive health risk. Hum Reprod Update. 2013;19:471-82.

Premature Ovarian Insufficiency

Rohan Palshetkar, Nandita Palshetkar, Jiteeka Thakkar

■ INTRODUCTION

Amenorrhea due to decreased ovarian function prior to the age of 40 years is known as premature ovarian insufficiency (POI). It can present either as primary amenorrhea prior to menarche or as secondary amenorrhea. It is a state of hypergonadotropic hypogonadism.

PREMATURE OVARIAN INSUFFICIENCY OR DIMINISHED OVARIAN RESERVE

Premature ovarian insufficiency and diminished ovarian reserve (DOR) go hand in hand even though there are separate situations presenting in different women with different treatment strategies.[1]

When we talk about ovarian reserve, it includes both the quality and quantity of the primordial follicles. In DOR patients, the ovarian reproductive potential is reduced.[1]

Ovarian stimulation in DOR patients results in a decreased number of oocytes retrieved. It also results in poor-quality blastocysts and therefore decreases the implantation potential of the embryos resulting in decreased clinical pregnancy rates (CPR).[2] About 9–24% of patients have DOR.[3] These patients have reduced anti-Müllerian hormone (AMH) due to a variety of reasons, but the most common cause is age.

DOR and POI must be distinguished even though they lie on a similar spectrum. This is due to POI patients facing a wider variety of health problems besides fertility which may require treatment.

■ PREVALENCE

Premature ovarian insufficiency is prevalent in 1% of the population. As mentioned above, there are a host of other medical issues associated with POI; therefore, factors such as smoking, surgical practice, and treatment regimens for malignant and chronic disease should be modified so as to reduce the iatrogenic risk for POI.[1]

■ SYMPTOMS

As a gynecologist, any woman with amenorrhea should be asked questions regarding symptoms such as:
- Menstrual abnormalities
- Sudden onset of secondary amenorrhea
- Vaginal dryness, hot flashes, sleep disturbances, mood changes, etc.
- Fertility history
- Hair loss
- Fatigue
- Anxiety/depression
- Altered urinary habits [recurrent urinary tract infection (UTI)]
- Low libido
- Lack of energy.

Women who present with POI at a younger age barely present with symptoms which suggest that the symptoms are due to estrogen withdrawal rather than deficiency, while patients with iatrogenic POI (bilateral oophorectomy) have severe persistent symptoms.[4]

■ CAUSES

The causes of premature ovarian insufficiency are as follows:
- *Spontaneous:*
  - Idiopathic
  - Genetic:
    - Turner syndrome (45,X0) or mosaic Turner (45,X/46,XX)
    - Trisomy X (47,XXX or mosaic)
    - Fragile X premutation
    - Galactosemia (galactose-1-phosphate uridylyltransferase deficiency)
    - Autoimmune polyglandular syndrome (types 1 and 2)
    - Follicle-stimulating hormone receptor mutations
    - 17α-hydroxylase deficiency
    - Aromatase deficiency
    - Blepharophimosis, ptosis, and epicanthus inversus syndrome
    - Bloom syndrome
    - Ataxia–telangiectasia
    - Fanconi anemia
  - Autoimmune
  - *Infections:*
    - Mumps oophoritis
    - Tuberculosis, malaria, cytomegalovirus, varicella, and shigella
- *Induced:*
  - Bilateral oophorectomy, bilateral ovarian cystectomies
  - Chemotherapy primarily, alkylating agents and anthracyclines

- Radiation—external beam or intracavitary
- Environmental toxins
- Pelvic vessel embolization.

■ DIAGNOSIS

Diagnostic considerations in evaluation of POI are given in **Table 1**. Diagnostic workup is given in **Table 2**.

■ GENETICS

The causative genes in POI are given in **Table 3**.

TABLE 1: Diagnostic considerations in evaluation of primary ovarian insufficiency.

Laboratory tests	Rationale
Human chorionic gonadotropins	Exclude pregnancy
• Follicle-stimulating hormone • Estradiol	Assess hypothalamic–pituitary–ovarian axis
Anti-Müllerian hormone	Assess ovarian reserve
Karyotype, fragile X mental retardation 1 (*FMR1*) premutation	Evaluate for genetic etiology
• Thyroid-stimulating hormone • Thyroid peroxidase antibody • 21-hydroxylase antibody	Thyroid function test. Check for dysfunction of thyroid and adrenal
Radiologic tests	**Rationale**
TVS (transvaginal ultrasound)	Evaluate antral follicle count to assess ovarian reserve
DEXA scan	Assess bone density

(DEXA: dual-energy X-ray absorptiometry)

TABLE 2: Summary of diagnostic workup.

Test	Positive test	Negative test
Genetic/chromosomal		
• Karyotyping for ruling out • Turner syndrome	Multidisciplinary approach with geneticist, endocrinologist, and cardiologist	A second analysis of the karyotype in epithelial cells (in case of high clinical suspicion)
Test for Y-chromosomal material	Counseling of patient for gonadectomy	
Fragile X syndrome	Consultation with geneticist	
Antibodies		
• ACA/21-OH antibodies • TPO-Ab	Endocrinology reference Annual thyroid function test	Repeat test in case of repeated symptoms

(ACA: anti-centromere antibody; 21-OH: 21-hydroxylase; TPO-Ab: thyroid peroxidase antibody)

TABLE 3: Causative genes in premature ovarian insufficiency (POI).

Gene	Mutation rate (%)	Functional category	Regulatory mechanism	Reference
LHX8	NA	Transcription factor	Germ-cell-specific critical regulator of early oogenesis	Rossetti et al. (2017)[5]
SOHLH1	NA	Transcription factor	Early folliculogenesis	Zhao et al. (2015)[6]
FOXO3A	2.2	Transcription factor	Regulating primordial follicle growth activation	Watkins et al. (2006)[7] John GB et al. (2008)[8]
NOBOX (7q35)	1.0–8.0	Transcription factor	Follicle development	Skillern A et al. (2004)[9]
FMR1 (Xq27)	0.5–6.7	Highly polymorphic CGG repeat in the 5′ untranslated region (UTR) of the exon 1	Transcriptional regulation	Brouwer JR (2009)[10]
PGRMC1 (Xq22-q24)	0.5–1.5	Heme-binding protein	Regulation of apoptosis	Venturella et al. (2019)[11]
POLR3H	1.5	RNA polymerase III subunit H	Regulation of cell cycle, cell growth, and differentiation	Franca et al. (2019)[12]
GDF9 (5q31.1)	0.5–4.7	Growth factor	Growth and differentiation of granulosa cell proliferation	Patiño et al. (2017)[13]
BMP15 (Xp11.2)	1.0–10.5	Growth factor	Growth and differentiation of granulosa cells (GCs)	di Pasquale et al. (2004)[14]
BMPR2	NA	BMP receptor	Signal transduction between oocytes and somatic cells	Patiño et al. (2017)[13]
AMH (19p13.3)	2.0	Anti-Müllerian hormone	Control of the formation of primary follicles by inhibiting excessive follicular recruitment by FSH	Alvaro Mercadal et al. (2015)[15]

Contd...

Contd...

Gene	Mutation rate (%)	Functional category	Regulatory mechanism	Reference
AMHR2 (12q13)	1.0–2.4	AMH receptor	AMH signal transduction	Yoon et al. (2013)[16]
FOXL2 (3q23)	1.0–2.9	Transcription factor	Differentiation and growth of granulosa cells	Bouilly et al. (2016)[17]
WT1 (11p13)	0.5	Transcription factor	Granulosa cell differentiation and oocyte–granulosa cell interaction	Gao et al. (2014)[18]
NR5A1 (9q33)	0.3–2.3	Transcription factor	Steroidogenesis in ovaries	Jiao et al. (2017)[19]
FSHR (2p21-p16)	0.1–42.3	Receptor	Follicular development and ovarian steroidogenesis	Welt et al. (2008)[20]
KHDRBS1	NA	Signal transduction activator	Alter mRNA expression level and alternative splicing	Wang et al. (2017)[21]
FIGLA (2p13.3)	0.5–2.0	bHLH transcription factor	Regulation of multiple oocyte-specific genes, including genes involved in folliculogenesis and those that encode the zona pellucida	Zhao et al. (2008)[22]
INHA variants	0–11	Growth factor	Maturation of ovarian follicles by FSH inhibition	Dixit et al. (2004)[23]
ESR1	NA	Estrogen receptor	Regulation of follicle growth and maturation and oocyte release	de Mattos et al. (2014)[24]
LHR	NA	Lutropin-choriogonadotropic hormone receptor	Regulation of ovarian follicle maturation, steroidogenesis, and ovulation	Simpson et al. (2008)[25]

(AMH: anti-Müllerian hormone; bHLH: basic helix–loop–helix; BMP: bone morphogenetic protein; FSH: follicle-stimulating hormone; mRNA: messenger RNA; NA: not applicable; RNA: ribonucleic acid)

WHAT IS THE CHANCE OF SPONTANEOUS PREGNANCY WITH A DIAGNOSIS OF PREMATURE OVARIAN INSUFFICIENCY?

Premature ovarian insufficiency patients may have ovarian activity; therefore, there is a possibility of natural pregnancy (5%). However, we must try and diagnose the cause for POI in patients with natural conception as it may have implications on the gestation and child (*FMR1* permutation).

ARE THERE TECHNIQUES AVAILABLE FOR FERTILITY PRESERVATION IN WOMEN WITH PREMATURE OVARIAN INSUFFICIENCY?

Fertility preservation (FP) may not be ideal in patients with POI as there is usually a loss of the ovarian reserve. But in some cases, there may be a window of opportunity, especially in the early course. In highly selective cases of Turner syndrome (adolescence and early adulthood), oocyte cryo-preservation or ovarian tissue cryopreservation (OTC) can be considered. Both these techniques have been reported; however, there have been no pregnancies post the procedures.[26-28]

Women at risk for POI should be considered candidates for FP. Survivors of childhood and adolescent cancers or sisters of women with POI are ideal candidates for FP. While the available biomarkers of ovarian reserve have some predictive value of time to menopause,[29,30] evidence linking reduced ovarian reserve in young women to fertility is very limited and indeed suggests that normal, regularly cycling women (mostly in their 20s) with low AMH levels do not have reduced fecundability.[31] But in patients aged 30–42 years, low AMH was associated with lower CPR.[32] Similarly, higher rates of spontaneous conception have been reported in women who underwent FP prior to their cancer treatments.[33]

■ TREATMENT FOR FERTILITY

Dehydroepiandrosterone

Dehydroepiandrosterone (DHEA) is a steroid which is formed in the adrenal cortex and theca cells of the ovary. It is a necessary prohormone in follicular steroidogenesis.[34] Therefore, supplementation of 75 mg daily for a minimum of 3 months is advised as it not only behaves like an antioxidant but also helps patients undergoing assisted reproductive technology (ART).

Coenzyme Q10

Coenzyme Q10 (CoQ10) is an antioxidant which helps in the body's production of adenosine triphosphate (ATP). It also helps in reducing lipid peroxidation and deoxyribonucleic acid (DNA) oxidation. Studies regarding

CoQ10 are conflicting with some cases suggesting improvement in fertility rates while others suggest its overall effect.[35]

Androgens: Testosterone Gel

As per the two-cell, two-gonadotropin theory, estrogen synthesis occurs in the granulosa cells while the precursor androgens are present in the theca cells. Androgen receptor expression can be found in the granulosa cells of the preantral and antral follicles. As the follicle matures, the expression decreases. This suggests that androgens play an important role in the early stages of maturation of the follicle. Many studies have concluded that androgens are very important for the recruitment and growth of the follicle. Furthermore, androgens induce the expression of micro-ribonucleic acid (RNA) miR-125b, which decreases the proapoptotic proteins. Androgens have also been found to induce follicle-stimulating hormone receptor (FSHR) messenger RNA (mRNA) expression during preantral to antral follicle progression. Whether this induction by androgens is mediated through androgen–androgen receptor (AR) response or by direct synergism between androgens and follicle stimulating hormone (FSH) in the ovary is not known. This suggests that androgen stimulation enhances follicular sensitivity toward FSH actions by increasing FSHR levels, which potentially contributes to follicle growth.[36,37] It has been suggested to apply 12.5 mg/day for 1–2 months prior to beginning ART treatment.

Oocyte Donation

Premature ovarian insufficiency patients will have the most success with oocyte donation (OD). The first successful case was reported in 1984.[38] Now, OD has become a part of routine practice. OD pregnancy rates are not greatly affected by the recipient's age.[39] Women with Turner syndrome have to be treated carefully as there are higher rates of complications in pregnancy and implantation.[40-42] Women with Turner syndrome have an increased chance of pregnancy loss, probably due to decreased endometrial and uterine function.[43]

WHAT ARE THE OBSTETRIC RISKS ASSOCIATED WITH PREMATURE OVARIAN INSUFFICIENCY?

Natural conception post idiopathic POI or cancer treatments usually have good outcome. Patients with pelvic irradiation may have increased obstetric risk due to decreased blood flow. Fertility also reduces post chemotherapy with alkylating agents.

Oocyte donation conceptions are at a higher risk of developing pregnancy-induced hypertension (PIH), undergoing lower segment cesarean section (LSCS) and postpartum hemorrhage (PPH). Intrauterine growth restriction (IUGR) is more common in women with OD conceptions. Therefore, it is recommended that OD patients should be categorized as high-risk pregnancies with detailed obstetric surveillance.[44]

The National Institute for Health and Care Excellence (NICE) guidelines have recommended that aspirin from 12 weeks' gestation should be given to women with risk of PIH. Since OD pregnancies have an increased risk of PIH, aspirin 75 mg should be started for these patients.

■ TREATMENT OF PREMATURE OVARIAN INSUFFICIENCY

Hormone Replacement Therapy

Hormone replacement therapy (HRT) has various routes of administration. The optimal method is to provide estrogen transdermally or through a vaginal ring. These routes have a lower risk of developing clots. Ideally, a combination of estrogen and progesterone is suggested; however, select cases can be given estrogen alone as well.[45,46]

Calcium and Vitamin D Supplements

Women with POI should receive 1,200–1,500 mg of calcium and 1,000 IU of vitamin D as they are at a higher risk of developing osteoporosis. Dual-energy X-ray absorptiometry (DEXA) scan must be done to check bone loss.[47]

▌RECENT ADVANCES IN THE MANAGEMENT OF PREMATURE OVARIAN INSUFFICIENCY (FIG. 1)

Currently used novel strategies mainly include:
- In vitro activation (IVA)
- Mitochondrial activation
- Stem cell and exosomes therapy
- Biomaterial strategies
- Intraovarian infusion of platelet-rich plasma (PRP).

These are all new novel techniques that are still in their experimental phase; therefore, their efficacy and safety must be proven prior to using them in daily clinical practice.

▌INNOVATIVE THERAPEUTIC OPTIONS FOR PREMATURE OVARIAN INSUFFICIENCY

In vitro Activation

A study has shown that 75% of patients with POI may have residual dormant primordial follicles.[48] The primordial follicles via IVA can be used to develop oocytes. By using this technique, the need for oocyte donors may be eliminated, and we will be able to provide the woman with an offspring with her own genetic material.

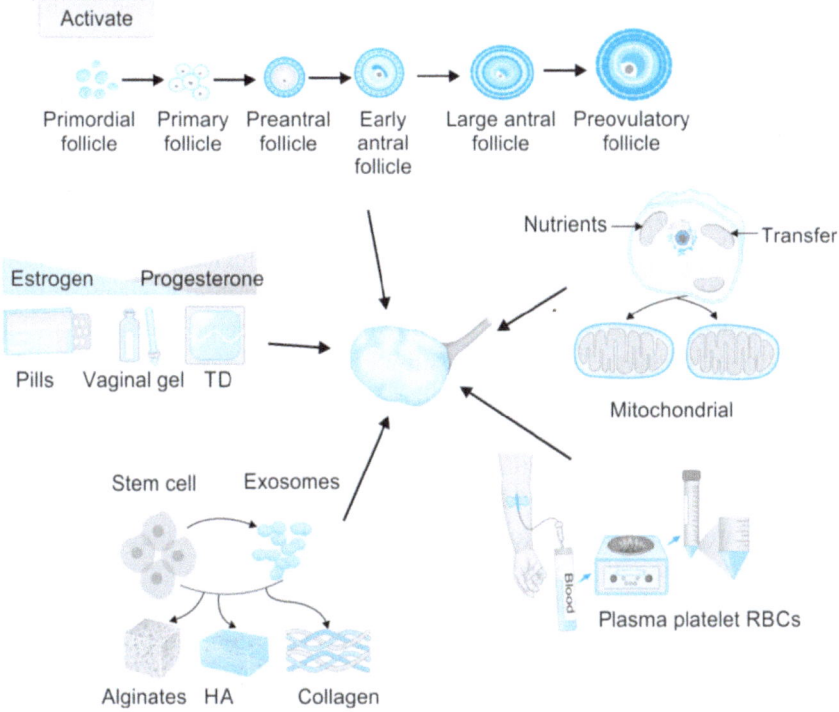

Fig. 1: Recent advances in the management of premature ovarian insufficiency. (HA: hyaluronic acid; RBC: red blood cell; TD: transdermal)

Ovarian tissue harvested laparoscopically is activated with phosphatase and tensin homolog (PTEN) inhibitors and phosphatidylinositol-3-kinase (PI3K) activators in an incubator. Following activation, the ovarian tissue is transplanted back into the ovarian fossa. There have been pregnancies that have been reported using the IVA technique.[40,49]

Drug-free IVA (new technique) works on the concept of disrupting the Hippo pathway and avoids chemical activation of ovaries. There has been an increased number of publications showing this technique to be successful in achieving pregnancies.[50-54]

Stem Cell Therapy

Stem cell therapy is expected to restore ovarian function and fertility for POI patients. Stem cells are early, undifferentiated cells with the ability to self-renew, unlimited proliferation, and multidifferentiation. They are classified as embryonic stem cells (ESCs), adult stem cells (ASCs), and induced pluripotent stem cells (iPSCs) according to their origin.[55] Mesenchymal stem cells (MSCs) are a subset of ASCs isolated from multiple tissues, including bone marrow, adipose tissue, menstrual blood, umbilical cord, amniotic fluid, and placenta.[56,57]

BIOMATERIAL STRATEGIES FOR PREMATURE OVARIAN INSUFFICIENCY

Stem cell transplantation leads to extreme cell loss. Consequently, biomaterials including collagen, alginate, and hyaluronic acid (HA) have to be introduced. Collagen is essential for maintaining biological activity. He et al. created collagen-rich, biomimetic 3D shells via microfluidic encapsulation, where follicle culture with these biomimetic capsules helped these to develop into the antral stage.[58] Su et al. used a collagen scaffold to enhance the retention of adipose-derived stem cells (ADSCs) in target organs.[59] Similarly, Ding et al. reported that umbilical cord mesenchymal stem cells (UC-MSCs) on collagen scaffolds activated follicles via the phosphorylation of FOXO3a and FOXO1.[60]

Alginates may be used for drug delivery due to their biocompatibility, nonimmunogenicity, and hydrophilicity. These have been used for the culture of secondary and preantral follicles.[61] ADSCs co-encapsulated with ovarian follicles in an alginate-based 3D culture system supported follicle genesis, survival, and maturation in vitro, via the secretion of cytokines.[62] HA is another widely used biological material. Certain tissues, such as those of the uterus and ovaries, that have HA receptors are amenable to targeted therapy.[63] Importantly, HA levels in POI patients are relatively low, and thus HA supplementation can be effectively used to prevent chemically induced ovarian injury and improve ovarian function.[64]

PLATELET-RICH PLASMA INTRAOVARIAN INFUSION

Mechanisms of Platelet-rich Plasma in Premature Ovarian Insufficiency

Premature ovarian insufficiency patients can benefit from intraovarian PRP. PRP is made of high concentration of platelets obtained from the blood of the patients.[65] PRP efficiency depends on the alpha granule, which is rich in protein, hormones, and growth factors.[66] PRP is said to improve cell proliferation and differentiation. In addition, there is angiogenesis along with anabolism and inflammation; therefore, repair of tissue occurs. Importantly, growth differentiation factor-9 (GDF-9), implicated in the maturation potential of oocytes and mutated in POI, is also present in PRP.[67-69]

It is still unclear how PRP works in patients of POI. There have been studies showing the benefits of PRP. It is said that PRP restores the ovarian microenvironment by reducing the oxidative stress on the ovary. PRP also reduces degeneration and atresia of normal follicles, which may have been caused by toxic chemicals.[70-74]

RISK AND COUNTERMEASURES OF PLATELET-RICH PLASMA THERAPY

The biggest advantage of PRP therapy is that it is autologous. In addition, the handling and storage properties make it easy to prepare and store. However, it does not come without its risks such as infection, intense cell proliferation, and unknown effects on the embryo.

Growth factors in PRP govern cell proliferation; however, an intense cell proliferation has a possibility of inducing malignancy due to the stem cells differentiating in the ovary. Infections are also associated with PRP, and these need to be detected and inactivated before PRP infusion.[66-80]

MICRO-RNA: THE FUTURE DIRECTION OF PREMATURE OVARIAN INSUFFICIENCY TREATMENT

Micro-ribonucleic acids (miRNAs) are short, 18–24 nucleotides long, non-coding RNAs. They are responsible for cell differentiation, proliferation, and apoptosis. miRNAs expression is linked with fertility potential and embryo development. They also have a regulatory role in the development of follicles as well as oocyte maturation. Currently, miRNAs are promising markers for cancers and other diseases.[81-83]

These novel treatment options will give all clinicians a chance to help their patients with POI conceive offspring with their own genetic material. Currently, the treatment has been OD for these patients, but the future looks promising, where the use of donor eggs may become a thing of the past.

KEY MESSAGES

- Ovarian activity is common in women with POI, especially early in the natural history of the condition.
- Most POI women had regular menses one year before diagnosis.
- Diagnostic testing includes:
  - Karyotype in all women with non-iatrogenic POI (Grade C)
  - FMR1 premutation testing (Grade B)
  - Autosomal genetic testing when evidence suggesting a specific mutation (GPP)
  - Steroidogenic cell autoantibodies (Grade C)
  - 21-hydroxylase autoantibodies and adrenal autoantibodies
  - Thyroid function studies with antibody testing (Grade C)
  - Transvaginal ultrasound
  - Bone mineral density
  - ACTH stimulation test as indicated.
- There are no known treatments which reliably increase ovulation rate, and the possibility of conception.
- Spontaneous pregnancy can occur in a small percentage of women.
- *Data from case series:* Lifetime chance of natural conception 4–5% after POI diagnosis with 80% of these pregnancies result in a live birth.

Contd...

Contd...

- In a subgroup of women, possibly with less advanced POI, estrogen treatment may increase the ovulation rate.
- Extremely difficult to establish criteria to define the population that should be treated and/or how to treat them.
- If follicles are present despite low ovarian reserve the treatment for fertility includes:
  - Start stimulation when baseline US shows sufficient number of follicles
  - Synchronize the follicle pool with premenstrual estrogen treatment or long protocol
  - Use a combination of FSH and LH
  - Dual stimulation or pooling when appropriate
  - No role for adjuvants (Androgens, DHEA or GH)
  - Embryo selection—transfer at the blastocyst stage, PGS, time lapse??
- Oocyte donation is the treatment of choice in women wishing to conceive.
- Innovative treatment options may pave the road to the future.
- *Newer Interventions:* Future potential solutions for low prognosis—in-vitro activation, mitochondrial transfer for gamete repair, stem cells, PRP, and pharmacogenomics.
- Fertility preservation may be advised if POI is detected early.
- However, these treatments should be tested rigorously first in animal models and then in randomized trials to prove their effectiveness and long-term safety.

■ REFERENCES

1. ESHRE Guideline Group on POI, Webber L, Davies M, Anderson R, Bartlett J, Braat D, Cartwright B, Cifkova R, de Muinck Keizer-Schrama S, Hogervorst E, Janse F. ESHRE Guideline: management of women with premature ovarian insufficiency. Human Reproduction. 2016;31(5):926-37.
2. Narkwichean A, Maalouf W, Campbell BK, Jayaprakasan K. Efficacy of dehydroepiandrosterone to improve ovarian response in women with diminished ovarian reserve: a meta-analysis. Reprod Biol Endocrinol. 2013;11:44.
3. Keay SD, Liversedge NH, Mathur RS, Jenkins JM. Assisted conception following poor ovarian response to gonadotrophin stimulation. Br J Obstet Gynaecol. 1997;104:521-7.
4. Rebar RW, Connolly HV. Clinical features of young women with hypergonadotropic amenorrhea. Fertil Steril. 1990;53:804-10.
5. Rossetti R, Ferrari I, Bonomi M, Persani L. Genetics of primary ovarian insufficiency. Clinical Genetics. 2017;91(2):183-98.
6. Zhao S, Li G, Dalgleish R, Vujovic S, Jiao X, Li J, Simpson JL, Qin Y, Ivanisevic M, Ivovic M, Tancic M. Transcription factor SOHLH1 potentially associated with primary ovarian insufficiency. Fertility and Sterility. 2015;103(2):548-53.
7. Watkins WJ, Umbers AJ, Woad KJ, Harris SE, Winship IM, Gersak K, Shelling AN. Mutational screening of FOXO3A and FOXO1A in women with premature ovarian failure. Fertility and Sterility. 2006;86(5):1518-21.
8. John GB, Gallardo TD, Shirley LJ, Castrillon DH. Foxo3 is a PI3K-dependent molecular switch controlling the initiation of oocyte growth. Developmental Biology. 2008;321(1):197-204.

9. Skillern A, Rajkovic A. Recent developments in identifying genetic determinants of premature ovarian failure. Sexual Development. 2008;2(4-5):228-43.
10. Brouwer JR, Willemsen R, Oostra BA. Microsatellite repeat instability and neurological disease. Bioessays. 2009;31(1):71-83.
11. Venturella R, De Vivo V, Carlea A, D'Alessandro P, Saccone G, Arduino B, Improda FP, Lico D, Rania E, De Marco C, Viglietto G. The genetics of non-syndromic primary ovarian insufficiency: a systematic review. International Journal of Fertility & Sterility. 2019;13(3):161.
12. Franca MM, Han X, Funari MF, Lerario AM, Nishi MY, Fontenele EG, Domenice S, Jorge AA, Garcia-Galiano D, Elias CF, Mendonca BB. Exome sequencing reveals the *POLR3H* gene as a novel cause of primary ovarian insufficiency. The Journal of Clinical Endocrinology & Metabolism. 2019;104(7):2827-41.
13. Patino LC, Beau I, Carlosama C, Buitrago JC, Gonzalez R, Suarez CF, Patarroyo MA, Delemer B, Young J, Binart N, et al. New mutations in non-syndromic primary ovarian insufficiency patients identified via whole-exome sequencing. Hum Reprod. 2017;32:1512-20.
14. Di Pasquale E, Beck-Peccoz P, Persani L. Hypergonadotropic ovarian failure associated with an inherited mutation of human bone morphogenetic protein-15 (*BMP15*) gene. The American Journal of Human Genetics. 2004;75(1):106-11.
15. Alvaro Mercadal B, Imbert R, Demeestere I, Gervy C, De Leener A, Englert Y, Costagliola S, Delbaere AJ. AMH mutations with reduced in vitro bioactivity are related to premature ovarian insufficiency. Human Reproduction. 2015;30(5):1196-202.
16. Yoon SH, Choi YM, Hong MA, Kim JJ, Lee GH, Hwang KR, Moon SY. Association study of anti-Müllerian hormone and anti-Müllerian hormone type II receptor polymorphisms with idiopathic primary ovarian insufficiency. Human Reproduction. 2013;28(12):3301-5.
17. Bouilly J, Beau I, Barraud S, Bernard V, Azibi K, Fagart J, Fevre A, Todeschini AL, Veitia RA, Beldjord C, et al. Identification of multiple gene mutations accounts for a new genetic architecture of primary ovarian insufficiency. J Clin Endocrinol Metab. 2016;101:4541-50.
18. Gao F, Zhang J, Wang X, Yang J, Chen D, Huff V, Liu YX. Wt1 functions in ovarian follicle development by regulating granulosa cell differentiation. Hum Mol Genet. 2014;23:333-41.
19. Jiao X, Zhang H, Ke H, Zhang J, Cheng L, Liu Y, Qin Y, Chen ZJ. Premature ovarian insufficiency: phenotypic characterization within different etiologies. The Journal of Clinical Endocrinology and Metabolism. 2017;102(7):2281-90.
20. Welt CK. Primary ovarian insufficiency: a more accurate term for premature ovarian failure. Clinical Endocrinology. 2008;68(4):499-509.
21. Wang B, Li L, Zhu Y, Zhang W, Wang X, Chen B, Li T, Pan H, Wang J, Kee K, Cao Y. Sequence variants of KHDRBS1 as high penetrance susceptibility risks for primary ovarian insufficiency by mis-regulating mRNA alternative splicing. Human Reproduction. 2017;32(10):2138-46.
22. Zhao H, Chen ZJ, Qin Y, Shi Y, Wang S, Choi Y, Simpson JL, Rajkovic A. Transcription factor FIGLA is mutated in patients with premature ovarian failure. The American Journal of Human Genetics. 2008;82(6):1342-8.

23. Dixit H, Rao KL, Padmalatha V, Kanakavalli M, Deenadayal M, Gupta N, Chakravarty BN, Singh L. Expansion of the germline analysis for the *INHA* gene in Indian women with ovarian failure. Human Reproduction. 2006;21(6):1643-4.
24. de Mattos CS, Trevisan CM, Peluso C, Adami F, Cordts EB, Christofolini DM, Barbosa CP, Bianco B. *ESR1* and *ESR2* gene polymorphisms are associated with human reproduction outcomes in Brazilian women. Journal of Ovarian Research. 2014;7(1):1-9.
25. Simpson JL. Genetic and phenotypic heterogeneity in ovarian failure: overview of selected candidate genes. Annals of the New York Academy of Sciences. 2008;1135(1):146-54.
26. Lau NM, Huang JY, MacDonald S, Elizur S, Gidoni Y, Holzer H, et al. Feasibility of fertility preservation in young females with Turner syndrome. Reprod Biomed Online. 2009;18:290-5.
27. Balen AH, Harris SE, Chambers EL, Picton HM. Conservation of fertility and oocyte genetics in a young woman with mosaic Turner syndrome. BJOG. 2010;117:238-42.
28. Borgstrom B, Hreinsson J, Rasmussen C, Sheikhi M, Fried G, Keros V, et al. Fertility preservation in girls with Turner syndrome: prognostic signs of the presence of ovarian follicles. J Clin Endocrinol Metab. 2009;94:74-80.
29. Broer SL, Eijkemans MJ, Scheffer GJ, van Rooij IA, de Vet A, Themmen AP, et al. Anti-Müllerian hormone predicts menopause: a long-term follow-up study in normoovulatory women. J Clin Endocrinol Metab. 2011;96:2532-9.
30. Freeman EW, Sammel MD, Lin H, Gracia CR. Anti-Müllerian hormone as a predictor of time to menopause in late reproductive age women. J Clin Endocrinol Metab. 2012;97:1673-80.
31. Hagen CP, Vestergaard S, Juul A, Skakkebaek NE, Andersson AM, Main KM, et al. Low concentration of circulating antimullerian hormone is not predictive of reduced fecundability in young healthy women: a prospective cohort study. Fertil Steril. 2012;98:1602-8.e2.
32. Steiner AZ, Herring AH, Kesner JS, Meadows JW, Stanczyk FZ, Hoberman S, et al. Anti-Müllerian hormone as a predictor of natural fecundability in women aged 30-42 years. Obstet Gynecol. 2011;117:798-804.
33. Schmidt KT, Nyboe Andersen A, Greve T, Ernst E, Loft A, Yding Andersen C. Fertility in cancer patients after cryopreservation of one ovary. Reprod Biomed Online. 2013;26:272-9.
34. Ozcil MD. Dehydroepiandrosterone supplementation improves ovarian reserve and pregnancy rates in poor responders. Eur Rev Med Pharmacol Sci. 2020;20:9104-11.
35. Showell MG, Mackenzie-Proctor R, Jordan V, Hart RJ. Antioxidants for female subfertility. Cochrane Database Syst Rev. 2017;7:CD007807.
36. Neves AR, Montoya-Botero P, Polyzos NP. The role of androgen supplementation in women with diminished ovarian reserve: time to randomize, not meta-analyze. Front Endocrinol (Lausanne). 2021;12:653857.
37. Mori T, Suzuki A, Nishimura T, Kambegawa A. Evidence for androgen participation in induced ovulation in immature rats. Endocrinology. 1977;101:623-6.
38. Lutjen P, Trounson A, Leeton J, Findlay J, Wood C, Renou P. The establishment and maintenance of pregnancy using in vitro fertilization and embryo donation in a patient with primary ovarian failure. Nature. 1984;307:174-5.

39. Templeton A, Morris JK, Parslow W. Factors that affect outcome of in-vitro fertilisation treatment. Lancet. 1996;348:1402-6.
40. Alvaro Mercadal B, Imbert R, Demeestere I, Englert Y, Delbaere A. Pregnancy outcome after oocyte donation in patients with Turner's syndrome and partial X monosomy. Hum Reprod. 2011;26:2061-8.
41. Foudila T, Soderstrom-Anttila V, Hovatta O. Turner's syndrome and pregnancies after oocyte donation. Hum Reprod. 1999;14:532-5.
42. Bodri D, Vernaeve V, Figueras F, Vidal R, Guillen JJ, Coll O. Oocyte donation in patients with Turner's syndrome: a successful technique but with an accompanying high risk of hypertensive disorders during pregnancy. Hum Reprod. 2006;21:829-32.
43. Bryman I, Sylven L, Berntorp K, Innala E, Bergstrom I, Hanson C, et al. Pregnancy rate and outcome in Swedish women with Turner syndrome. Fertil Steril. 2011;95:2507-10.
44. Stoop D, Baumgarten M, Haentjens P, Polyzos NP, De Vos M, Verheyen G, et al. Obstetric outcome in donor oocyte pregnancies: a matched-pair analysis. Reprod Biol Endocrinol. 2012;10:42.
45. Kodaman PH. Early menopause: primary ovarian insufficiency and surgical menopause. Semin Reprod Med. 2010;28:360-9.
46. National Library of Medicine, MedlinePlus. (2010). Estrogen vaginal. [online] Available from https://medlineplus.gov/druginfo/meds/a606005.html [Last accessed November, 2022].
47. Institute of Medicine of the National Academies. In: Ross AC, Taylor CL, Yaktine AL, Del Valle HB (Eds). Dietary Reference Intakes for Calcium and Vitamin D. Washington: National Academies Press (US); 2011.
48. De Vos M, Devroey P, Fauser BC. Primary ovarian insufficiency. Lancet. 2010;376:911-21.
49. Zhai J, Yao G, Dong F, Bu Z, Cheng Y, Sato Y, et al. In vitro activation of follicles and fresh tissue auto-transplantation in primary ovarian insufficiency patients. J Clin Endocrinol Metab. 2016;101:4405-12.
50. Kawamura K, Ishizuka B, Hsueh AJW. Drug-free in-vitro activation of follicles for infertility treatment in poor ovarian response patients with decreased ovarian reserve. Reprod Biomed Online. 2020;40:245-53.
51. Ferreri J, Fabregues F, Calafell JM, Solernou R, Borras A, Saco A, et al. Drug-free in-vitro activation of follicles and fresh tissue autotransplantation as a therapeutic option in patients with primary ovarian insufficiency. Reprod Biomed Online. 2020;40:254-60.
52. Resetkova N, Hayashi M, Kolp LA, Christianson MS. Fertility preservation for prepubertal girls: update and current challenges. Curr Obstet Gynecol Rep. 2013;2:218-25.
53. De Roo C, Lierman S, Tilleman K, De Sutter P. In-vitro fragmentation of ovarian tissue activates primordial follicles through the Hippo pathway. Hum Reprod Open. 2020;2020:hoaa048.
54. Gavish Z, Spector I, Peer G, Schlatt S, Wistuba J, Roness H, et al. Follicle activation is a significant and immediate cause of follicle loss after ovarian tissue transplantation. J Assist Reprod Genet. 2018;35:61-9.
55. Kolios G, Moodley Y. Introduction to stem cells and regenerative medicine. Respiration. 2012;85:3-10.

56. Na J, Kim GJ. Recent trends in stem cell therapy for premature ovarian insufficiency and its therapeutic potential: a review. J Ovarian Res. 2020;13:74.
57. Chen L, Qu J, Xiang C. The multi-functional roles of menstrual blood-derived stem cells in regenerative medicine. Stem Cell Res Ther. 2019;10:1.
58. He X. Microfluidic encapsulation of ovarian follicles for 3D culture. Ann Biomed Eng. 2017;45:1676-84.
59. Su J, Ding L, Cheng J, Yang J, Li X, Yan G, et al. Transplantation of adipose-derived stem cells combined with collagen scaffolds restores ovarian function in a rat model of premature ovarian insufficiency. Hum Reprod. 2016;31:1075-86.
60. Ding L, Yan G, Wang B, Xu L, Gu Y, Ru T, et al. Transplantation of UC-MSCs on collagen scaffold activates follicles in dormant ovaries of POF patients with long history of infertility. Sci China Life Sci. 2018;61:1554-65.
61. Amorim CA, Van Langendonckt A, David A, Dolmans MM, Donnez J. Survival of human pre-antral follicles after cryopreservation of ovarian tissue, follicular isolation and in vitro culture in a calcium alginate matrix. Hum Reprod. 2009;24:92-9.
62. Green LJ, Zhou H, Padmanabhan V, Shikanov A. Adipose-derived stem cells promote survival, growth, and maturation of early-stage murine follicles. Stem Cell Res Ther. 2019;10:102.
63. Kim H, Shin M, Han S, Kwon W, Hahn SK. Hyaluronic acid derivatives for translational medicines. Biomacromolecules. 2019;20:2889-903.
64. Zhao G, Zhou X, Fang T, Hou Y, Hu Y. Hyaluronic acid promotes the expression of progesterone receptor membrane component 1 via epigenetic silencing of miR-139-5p in human and rat granulosa cells. Biol Reprod. 2014;91:116.
65. Bos-Mikich A, de Oliveira R, Frantz N. Platelet-rich plasma therapy and reproductive medicine. J Assist Reprod Genet. 2018;35:753-6.
66. Sfakianoudis K, Simopoulou M, Grigoriadis S, Pantou A, Tsioulou P, Maziotis E, et al. Reactivating ovarian function through autologous platelet-rich plasma intraovarian infusion: pilot data on premature ovarian insufficiency, perimenopausal, menopausal, and poor responder women. J Clin Med. 2020;9:1809.
67. Sundman EA, Cole BJ, Karas V, Della Valle C, Tetreault MW, Mohammed HO, et al. The anti-inflammatory and matrix restorative mechanisms of platelet-rich plasma in osteoarthritis. Am J Sports Med. 2014;42:35-41.
68. Cakiroglu Y, Saltik A, Yuceturk A, Karaosmanoglu O, Kopuk SY, Scott RT, et al. Effects of intraovarian injection of autologous platelet rich plasma on ovarian reserve and IVF outcome parameters in women with primary ovarian insufficiency. Aging. 2020;12:10211-22.
69. Sfakianoudis K, Simopoulou M, Nitsos N, Rapani A, Pappas A, Pantou A, et al. Autologous platelet-rich plasma treatment enables pregnancy for a woman in premature menopause. J Clin Med. 2018;8:1.
70. Hosseini L, Shirazi A, Naderi MM, Shams-Esfandabadi N, Borjian Boroujeni S, Sarvari A, et al. Platelet-rich plasma promotes the development of isolated human primordial and primary follicles to the preantral stage. Reprod Biomed Online. 2017;35:343-50.
71. Jeppesen JV, Anderson RA, Kelsey TW, Christiansen SL, Kristensen SG, Jayaprakasan K, et al. Which follicles make the most anti-mullerian hormone

in humans? Evidence for an abrupt decline in AMH production at the time of follicle selection. Mol Hum Reprod. 2013;19:519-27.
72. Gracia CR, Shin SS, Prewitt M, Chamberlin JS, Lofaro LR, Jones KL, et al. Multicenter clinical evaluation of the access AMH assay to determine AMH levels in reproductive age women during normal menstrual cycles. J Assist Reprod Genet. 2018;35:777-83.
73. Bakacak M, Bostanci MS, Inanc F, Yaylali A, Serin S, Attar R, et al. Protective effect of platelet rich plasma on experimental ischemia/reperfusion injury in rat ovary. Gynecol Obstet Investig. 2016;81:225-31.
74. Ahmadian S, Sheshpari S, Pazhang M, Bedate AM, Beheshti R, Abbasi MM, et al. Intra-ovarian injection of platelet-rich plasma into ovarian tissue promoted rejuvenation in the rat model of premature ovarian insufficiency and restored ovulation rate via angiogenesis modulation. Reprod Biol Endocrinol. 2020;18:78.
75. Pantos K, Nitsos N, Kokkali G, Vaxevanoglou T, Markomichali C, Pantou A, et al. Ovarian rejuvenation and folliculogenesis reactivation in perimenopausal women after autologous platelet-rich plasma treatment. Hum Reprod. 2016;(Suppl. 1):i301.
76. Callejo J, Salvador C, Gonzalez-Nunez S, Almeida L, Rodriguez L, Marques L, et al. Live birth in a woman without ovaries after autograft of frozen-thawed ovarian tissue combined with growth factors. J Ovarian Res. 2013;6:33.
77. Hsu CC, Hsu L, Hsu I, Chiu YJ, Dorjee S. Live birth in woman with premature ovarian insufficiency receiving ovarian administration of platelet-rich plasma (PRP) in combination with gonadotropin: a case report. Front Endocrinol (Lausanne). 2020;11:50.
78. Reurink G, Goudswaard GJ, Moen MH, Weir A, Verhaar JAN, Bierma-Zeinstra SMA, et al. Rationale, secondary outcome scores and 1-year follow-up of a randomised trial of platelet-rich plasma injections in acute hamstring muscle injury: the Dutch Hamstring Injection Therapy study. Br J Sports Med. 2015;49:1206-12.
79. Schepull T, Kvist J, Norrman H, Trinks M, Berlin G, Aspenberg P. Autologous platelets have no effect on the healing of human Achilles tendon ruptures: a randomized single-blind study. Am J Sports Med. 2011;39:38-47.
80. Scott Sills E, Wood SH. Autologous activated platelet-rich plasma injection into adult human ovary tissue: molecular mechanism, analysis, and discussion of reproductive response. Biosci Rep. 2019;39:BSR20190805.
81. Zhang J, Xu Y, Liu H, Pan Z. MicroRNAs in ovarian follicular atresia and granulosa cell apoptosis. Reprod Biol Endocrinol. 2019;17:9.
82. Imbar T, Eisenberg I. Regulatory role of microRNAs in ovarian function. Fertil Steril. 2014;101:1524-30.
83. Salas-Huetos A, James ER, Aston KI, Jenkins TG, Carrell DT, Yeste M. The expression of miRNAs in human ovaries, oocytes, extracellular vesicles, and early embryos: a systematic review. Cells. 2019;8:1564.

Aging Ovary

Madhuri Patil, Archana Baser, Anshu Baser

■ INTRODUCTION

The ovary is responsible for periodic release of gametes and the production of the female steroid hormones estradiol and progesterone. This is a result of cyclic follicle maturation, ovulation, and corpus luteum formation and regression. Ovarian aging is characterized by gradual decline in ovarian follicle quantity and quality, ending with menopause. The ovarian aging process is complicated and affected by a number of factors, including lifestyle, exposure to medicines, genetic, autoimmune, environmental, and idiopathic ones. Ovarian aging is already quite advanced when the first clinical sign appears as menstrual cycles remain regular, though overall cycle length and variability decrease gradually.

The germ cells are first identified at the end of the 3rd week after fertilization in the primitive endoderm at the caudal end in the dorsal wall of the adjacent yolk sac, and, soon, they also appear in the splanchnic mesoderm of and "migrate" from the yolk sac around the hindgut to their gonadal sites between 4 and 6 weeks of gestation.[1,2] At 6-8 weeks, the first signs of ovarian differentiation are seen with rapid mitotic multiplication of germ cells, reaching 6-7 million by 16-20 weeks.[3,4] This is the maximal oogonal content of the gonad ever. From here on, the germ cell number will irretrievably decrease until 45-50 years later, when the store of oocytes/germ cells will be finally exhausted **(Fig. 1)**. In the second half of pregnancy with follicular growth and atresia, there is a substantial decrease in the number of oocytes during meiosis, and those oogonia that fail to be enveloped by granulosa cells also undergo degeneration. This process of follicular or germ cell loss is influenced by genes.[5] The ovary at birth contains primordial follicle—an oocyte arrested in prophase of meiosis, enveloped by a single layer of spindle-shaped pregranulosa cells, surrounded by a basement membrane. The number of germ cells reduces to 1-2 million by birth as a result of prenatal oocyte depletion over a short period of 20 weeks.[6] Because of the fixed initial number of germ cells, the newborn female enters life, with having lost 80% of her oocytes. At the onset of puberty, the germ cell number is reduced further to 300,000-400,000.[4,7] During the next 35-40 years

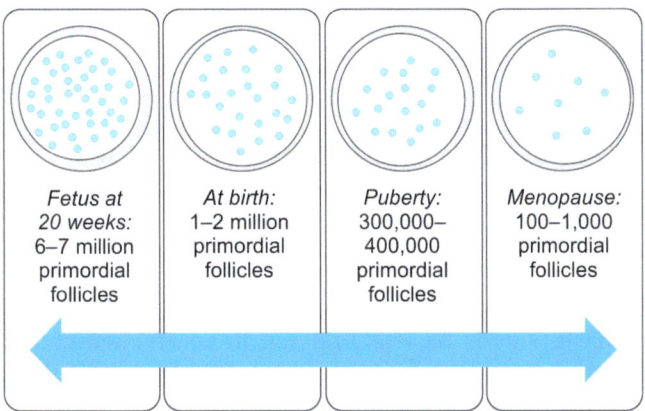

Fig. 1: Primordial follicles from in utero to menopause.

of reproductive life, 400–500 primordial follicles will be selected to grow and ovulate. The primordial follicles will eventually be depleted to a few hundred to a thousand at menopause.[5,8-10]

Thus, with age, there is depletion of the number of primordial follicles and the age of menopause is determined by the rate at which follicles deplete. With follicular depletion, the ovarian reserve decreases and so also fertility.[10-12] There is a gradual increase in the rate of follicular depletion, and this increases further as the number of follicles remaining decreases. This is probably related to a decrease in paracrine factors secreted by primordial follicles, which inhibit recruitment and regulate the size of the resting follicular pool.[13-15] Overall, fertility rates are 4–8% lower in women aged 25–29 years, 15–19% lower in those aged 30–34 years, 26–46% lower in women aged 35–39 years, and as much as 95% lower for women aged 40–45 years.[16,17]

There could be variations in fertility rates at different ages depending on genetic factors, socioeconomic conditions, ethnicity, and presence of polycystic ovary syndrome (PCOS).

The rate of decline of follicles depends on:
- Follicle reserve at birth
- Rate of follicle depletion
- Rate at which follicles enter growing pool
  - Too high
  - Too low
- Rate of atresia.

It is the programmed cell death that determines the time of ovarian depletion, thus the follicular pool at any time. Human mural luteinized granulosa cells exhibit a reduction in their energy metabolism as women age that is likely to influence female reproductive potential.[18] It has been seen that age-related loss of fertility precedes the menopause by ~12 years.

Approximately 10% of women enter the menopause in their early 40s and approximately 1% of women enter the menopause in their 30s which may be related to starting off with fewer eggs.

■ ENDOCRINOLOGY OF REPRODUCTIVE AGING

With ovarian aging, serum follicle-stimulating hormone (FSH) levels begin to rise, though the luteinizing hormone (LH) concentrations remain unchanged. The increase in FSH is observed more in the intermenstrual cycle phase at the end of luteal phase and just before beginning of the follicular phase. This is basically related to age-related changes in the pattern of pulsatile kisspeptin and gonadotropin-releasing hormone (GnRH) secretion or from progressive follicular depletion and decreased inhibitory feedback by ovarian hormones.[19] Circulating follicular phase inhibin B levels decrease as or even before FSH concentrations begin to increase.[20-24] Inhibin A levels also decrease, but only in the later stages of ovarian/reproductive aging, and is mostly seen after the onset of menstrual irregularity.[25-27] Follicular phase estradiol levels in older cycling women are generally even higher than young women[28,29] whereas luteal phase estrogen and progesterone levels may be lower with advancing age unless the women has an occasional ovulatory cycle.[21,30-32] As the follicular phase shortens with increased FSH levels, estradiol levels rise earlier. This may be due to higher FSH levels that stimulate more rapid follicular development.[33] The menopausal transition begins at an average age of 46 years, but can vary and can be as early as 34 years and as late as 54 years.[34-36] During menopausal transition, the average cycle length and variability increase steadily as ovulations become less regular and frequent.[37] Regardless of age, the interval from loss of menstrual regularity to menopause is relatively fixed, spanning approximately 5–6 years.[35,38] The average age of menopause is usually 51 years but may range between the ages of 40 and 60 years.[39]

■ AGING FOLLICLE AND OOCYTE

With ovarian aging apart from decrease in follicular number, the quality of the oocyte also deteriorates. This may be related to an increase in meiotic non-disjunction, resulting in an increasing rate of oocyte and embryo aneuploidy in aging women.[40-42] This increase in oocyte and embryo aneuploidy is primarily the cause of decrease in fecundability and increase in the incidence of miscarriage.

In controlled ovarian stimulation (COS) cycles, it was seen that aging follicles also become progressively less sensitive to gonadotropin stimulation and therefore require a higher total dose of gonadotropins and require an increased duration of treatment to stimulate multiple follicular development. The rate of rise and the peak in estradiol levels decrease, suggesting that a smaller cohort of follicles been recruited. However, the amount of estradiol secreted by the dominant follicles which grow to maturity is comparable to that in younger women.[43]

■ EARLY OVARIAN AGING

This concept was initially proposed by Nikolaou and Templeton in 2003 and is experienced by around 10% of women.[44] It implies a condition in which there is a low ovarian reserve at an earlier age and expedited loss of ovarian follicles in the early thirties. These women routinely have regular cycles and are asymptomatic. As the condition progresses, it leads to irregular menses, decline of fertility, and finally menopause. Early ovarian aging (EOA) is, therefore, the asymptomatic predecessor of early menopause or, at the farthest end of the ovarian aging spectrum, premature ovarian insufficiency (POI)/premature menopause **(Table 1)**. It has, however, been found that in women with this condition, the oocyte number is lost more promptly than oocyte quality and therefore these women will have good fertility outcomes when they are young.

Etiology of Early Ovarian Aging

The main risk factors for early ovarian aging are as follows **(Fig. 2)**:
- *Genetic:* A family history of premature menopause; x chromosome derangements: mosaics, deletions, inversions and translocations; FMR1 (fragile x) gene; gene polymorphisms of anti-Müllerian hormone (AMH) and AMH receptor genes and trisomy 21
- *Autoimmune factors:* Thyroid autoimmunity, autoimmune oophoritis
- *Acquired modifiable factors:* Chemotherapy, radiotherapy, pelvic surgery, pelvic infections or tubal disease, severe endometriosis, and heavy smoking.

Young women with EOA are not infertile though have a reduced fertility potential. They may take longer to conceive or present with

TABLE 1: A comparison of early ovarian aging and premature ovarian insufficiency.

Early ovarian aging	Premature ovarian insufficiency
10% prevalence	1% prevalence
Regular periods	Oligomenorrhea or amenorrhea
Asymptomatic	Other symptoms of estrogen deficiency may coexist
FSH normal or mildly elevated	FSH markedly elevated (>25–30 IU/L)
ERT not advised	ERT advised
Fertility preserved until late	Spontaneous conception <5%

(ERT: estrogen replacement therapy; FSH: follicle-stimulating hormone)

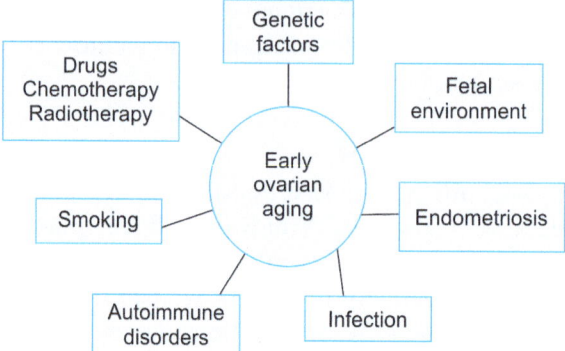

Fig. 2: Risk factors for early ovarian aging.

unexplained infertility. EOA also results in rapid decline in pregnancy rates both naturally and with in vitro fertilization (IVF) and is related to decline in the oocyte quality along with quantity.[45] During IVF cycles, they may behave as poor responders to COS and will require higher doses of gonadotropins. There is also an increase in the rate of spontaneous miscarriages and chromosomal abnormalities in the embryos.[45] The main cause of deterioration of oocyte quality is meiotic nondisjunction.[46] Elevated FSH concentration in the early follicular phase has been shown to be associated with trisomy 21 and other aneuploidies.[47]

Patients with accelerated aging syndromes such as Werner syndrome, ataxia telangiectasia, Hutchison–Gilford progeria, and Down syndrome are either infertile or have an early menopause.[48] An association has also been seen between early menopause and shorter life expectancy.[49]

Consequences of Ovarian Aging

With age, as FSH increases the follicular phase is shorter, the dominant follicle identified earlier due to high pre-/intermenstrual FSH levels and the diameter of dominant follicle before ovulation is much smaller which could be an indicator of diminished follicle quality.[50,51] Whether the dominant follicle has an accelerated or advance growth is debatable. Usually, the LH levels and luteal phase duration remain unchanged. With aging, there is a decrease in androgen levels [total and free testosterone, dehydroepiandrosterone sulfate (DHEAS) and androstenedione] which may be related to less function; LH receptors and endogenous LH may be less potent and biologically active or there could be impaired ovarian paracrine activity.[52]

Women with advanced age had a lower rate of spontaneous conception and also had an increased time to pregnancy. Moreover, the pregnancy was associated with a higher incidence of medical complications and more interventions during labor.[53] The earlier increase in follicular phase FSH level frequently results in more than one dominant follicle growing which may be the cause of a higher prevalence of dizygotic twinning in older cycling women.[54,55] The miscarriage rate also increases with ovarian aging.[56,57]

Assisted reproductive technology (ART) was not a panacea for subfertility associated with aging. Success rates achieved with ART using self-eggs also decline with age. The numbers of oocytes retrieved and embryos available for transfer, implantation rate, pregnancy rate, and live birth rates were all lower in older than in younger women.[58] Moreover, cost per live birth from IVF increases with maternal age and order of attempts. Thus, the cost for treating old IVF patients need to be considered in counseling these patients.[59]

Age, antral follicle count (AFC), and AMH significantly correlated with clinical pregnancy rate though AFC had the highest accuracy. The optimum cutoff value of age was ≤41, that of AFC was >3, and that of the number of total retrieved oocytes was >6 to predict clinical pregnancy.[60] The other factors that can predict live birth rate are number of previous cycles, number of oocytes retrieved, number of good-quality embryos on day 2, number of transferred embryos, proportion of blastocyst transfer, and number of frozen blastocysts.[60] The more embryos transferred, the higher the probability of live birth in patients >40 years of age; however, twins and triplets are still possible. The availability of embryos for cryopreservation after a fresh transfer is associated with a significantly higher probability of live birth in patients >40 years of age. Despite a higher oocyte yield in all age groups, women with PCOS over the age of 40 years had similar cumulative pregnancy rate (CPR) and live birth rate (LBR) when compared to women with tubal factor infertility. Thus, the reproductive window may not be extended in PCOS and that patients with infertility should be treated in a timely manner despite indicators of high ovarian reserve.[61]

Screening

There is at present no fixed screening protocol for these women. However, screening would involve tests for ovarian reserve assessment, which could be basal endocrine assays (FSH, AMH), biophysical tests (AFC and ovarian volume) **(Figs. 3 and 4)**, ovarian biopsies, and the IVF procedure itself.

Although AFC is easy to evaluate and easily accessible to all patients, there are many issues such as patient acceptability and intercycle and interobserver variability. It could be used early in women with subfertility, poor responders to stimulation, history of early/premature menopause in other members of the family, surgical history for treatment of cancer or ovarian surgery, and history of chemotherapy or radiotherapy. If EOA is diagnosed, these women can plan parenthood at an earlier age, and this can significantly improve their reproductive outcomes.

For women in POSEIDON groups 1, 2, and 3, the prognosis was favorable after three successive cycles of IVF/intracytoplasmic sperm

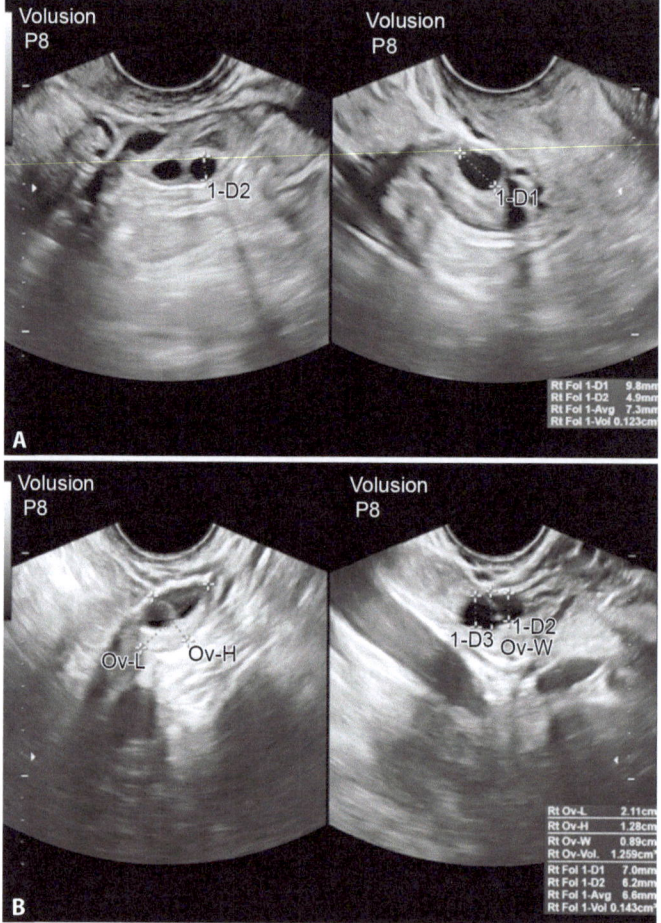

Figs. 3A and B: Low antral follicle count.

injection (ICSI) treatment. POSEIDON group 4 in women with old age and decreased ovarian reserve (DOR) had poor prognosis. Higher LBR was observed in younger patients (POSEIDON groups 1 and 3) than older patients (POSEIDON groups 2 and 4) in the subgroup analysis ($p < 0.001$).[62]

TREATMENT FOR FERTILITY IN WOMEN WITH AGING OVARIES

It is extremely difficult to establish criteria to define the population that should be treated and/or how to treat them. All types of empirical interventions are being tried, some with a hypothesis behind them, which might be biologically plausible, others with less plausibility.

Table 2 gives the evidence for use of different treatment strategies in women with aging ovaries. Most of the treatment modalities used do not

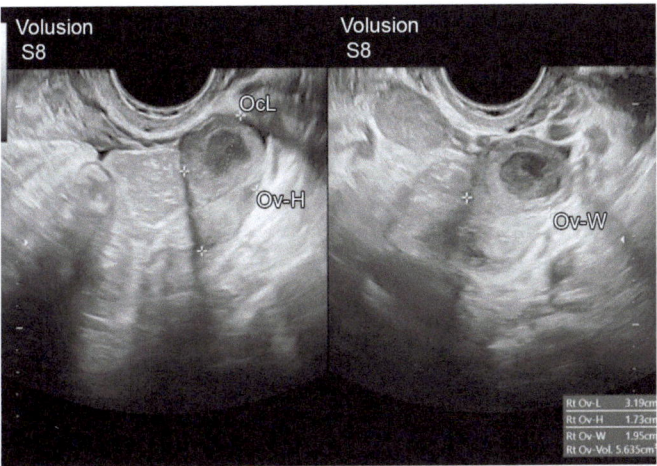

Fig. 4: Low ovarian volume.

TABLE 2: Treatment strategies in women with aging ovaries.

Strategy	Live birth rate
Change protocol (agonist vs. antagonist vs. microdose, letrozole)	No difference
Change gonadotropin (hMG vs. rFSH)	No difference
Add LH/hCG	More data needed—effect most likely marginal
Prime with androgens	More data needed—effect most likely marginal
Growth hormone	No difference
Dual stimulation	No data
Natural cycle	No difference
Oocyte donation	Proven efficacy

(hCG: human chorionic gonadotropin; hMG: human menopausal gonadotropin; LH: luteinizing hormone; rFSH: recombinant follicle-stimulating hormone)

have much evidence and have not helped in increasing the pregnancy rates in women with aged ovaries.

■ PREVENTION STRATEGIES, PUBLIC AWARENESS

Primary prevention: Avoid smoking, pelvic infection, and ablative and definitive surgical interventions. One should also avoid postponing childbearing to advanced age.

It requires detailed counseling, and all women should be informed that fertility declines with age and this should be emphasized. It should be emphasized that these women are fertile when they are asymptomatic and have regular cycles. A complete picture about reproductive health and general health consequences should be given to these women. Information can improve their autonomy and reproductive outcomes.

ETHICAL ISSUES

Two main ethical issues when it comes to ovarian aging, especially EOA, are:
1. Should women be screened for EOA?
2. What is the efficacy of egg freezing for fertility preservation?

We still do not have an answer for it.

CONCLUSION

Natural fertility normally declines with maternal age, which is related to ovarian follicle depletion. In a normal woman, an accelerated decline in fertility is seen in the late thirties. Most of the decline in natural fertility with age is caused by decreasing oocyte quality and an increasing risk of early pregnancy loss, which may be related to aneuploidy. Ovarian reserve tests such as basal endocrine assays, biophysical tests, ovarian biopsies, and the IVF procedure itself will identify patients with early ovarian aging. A detailed counseling will help in starting appropriate treatment early, with an optimal outcome. The probability of live birth in women >40 years of age is small and decreases significantly with each additional year. Certain interventions are associated with a small increase in ovarian response, the clinical significance of which, however, is debatable. One must also remember that the obstetric risks also increase in women with advanced maternal age with both natural and IVF conceptions.

KEY MESSAGES

- The cause of declining fertility in elderly women with a regular menstrual cycle is not clear, but may be due to a higher incidence of subtle cycle disorders such as anovulatory cycles, hormonal changes, diminished uterine receptivity, and oocyte factor.
- There is no specification for an upper age limit for treatment. Clinics make their own determinations about patients.
- In older women, with age there is a decline in ovarian reserve and follicular recruitment and number of oocytes collected and an increase in daily and total FSH dose required with increased days of stimulation and physical and emotional stress.
- To predict the live birth, age ≤41 years, AFC >3, and total retrieved oocytes >6 appeared to be meaningful.
- EOA affects around 10% of women.
- Women with early ovarian aging are frequently asymptomatic with normal fertility; however, continuing follicular loss will result in loss of fertility, menstrual irregularity, and, finally, early menopause.

Contd…

Contd...

- As women increasingly delay childbirth, the physical, psychological, and financial impact of EOA is escalating.
- Long-term health effects include early menopause and increased cardiovascular risk.
- Improvements in the success of oocyte freezing have provided a treatment option when EOA is identified early.
- Autologous IVF carries a low success rate and a considerable risk of decision regret in women >42 years of age.
- In those who were unsuccessful, the perceived adequacy of information and that of emotional support were protective factors against increased regret.
- Short-term and long-term emotional support when providing treatment to this patient group will help to decrease their level of long-term regret.
- Ample counseling and psychological support should be particularly emphasized within this patient population.
- If there are no visible follicles, success is unlikely as unfortunately one cannot recruit or stimulate what is not there and egg quality fundamentally cannot be altered.

REFERENCES

1. Pereda M, Zorn T, Soto-Suazo M. Migration of human and mouse primordial germ cells and colonization of the developing ovary: an ultrastructural and cytochemical study. Microsc Res Tech. 2006;69:386-95.
2. Motta PM, Nottola SA, Makabe S. Natural history of the female germ cell from its origin to full maturation through prenatal ovarian development. Eur J Obstet Gynecol Reprod Biol. 1997;75:5-10.
3. Baker TG. A quantitative and cytological study of germ cells in human ovaries. Proc R Soc Lond B Biol Sci. 1963;158:417-33.
4. Gondos B, Bhiraleus P, Hobel CJ. Ultrastructural observations on germ cells in human fetal ovaries. Am J Obstet Gynecol. 1971;110:644-52.
5. Richardson SJ, Senikas V, Nelson JF. Follicular depletion during the menopausal transition: evidence for accelerated loss and ultimate exhaustion. J Clin Endocrinol Metab. 1987;65:1231.
6. Markström E, Svensson ECh, Shao R, Svanberg B, Billig H. Survival factors regulating ovarian apoptosis—dependence on follicle differentiation. Reproduction. 2002;123:23-30.
7. te Velde ER, Pearson PL. The variability of female reproductive ageing. Hum Reprod Update. 2002;8:141-54.
8. Faddy MJ, Gosden RG. A model conforming the decline in follicle numbers to the age of menopause in women. Hum Reprod. 1996;11:1484-6.
9. Battaglia DE, Goodwin P, Klein NA, Soules MR. Influence of maternal age on meiotic spindle assembly in oocytes from naturally cycling women. Hum Reprod. 1996;11:2217-22.
10. Gougeon A, Ecochard R, Thalabard JC. Age-related changes of the population of human ovarian follicles: increase in the disappearance rate of non-growing and early-growing follicles in aging women. Biol Reprod. 1994;50:653-63.
11. Block E. Quantitative morphological investigations of the follicular system in women; variations at different ages. Acta Anat (Basel). 1952;14:108-23.

12. Faddy MJ, Gosden RG, Gougeon A, Richardson SJ, Nelson JF. Accelerated disappearance of ovarian follicles in mid-life: implications for forecasting menopause. Hum Reprod. 1992;7:1342-6.
13. Himelstein-Braw R, Byskov AG, Peters H, Faber M. Follicular atresia in the infant human ovary. J Reprod Fertil. 1976;46:55-9.
14. Forabosco A, Sforza C, De Pol A, Vizzotto L, Marzona L, Ferrario VF. Morphometric study of the human neonatal ovary. Anat Rec. 1991;231:201-8.
15. Forabosco A, Sforza C. Establishment of ovarian reserve: a quantitative morphometric study of the developing human ovary. Fertil Steril. 2007;88:675-83.
16. Maroulis GB. Effect of Aging on Fertility and Pregnancy. Semin Reprod Endocrinol. 1991;9:165-75.
17. van Noord-Zaadstra BM, Looman CW, Alsbach H, Habbema JD, te Velde ER, Karbaat J. Delaying childbearing: effect of age on fecundity and outcome of pregnancy. BMJ. 1991;302:1361-5.
18. Cecchino GN, García-Velasco JA, Rial E. Reproductive senescence impairs the energy metabolism of human luteinized granulosa cells. Reprod Biomed Online. 2021;43(5):779-87.
19. Burger HG, Dudley EC, Hopper JL, Groome N, Guthrie JR, Green A, et al. Prospectively measured levels of serum follicle-stimulating hormone, estradiol, and the dimeric inhibins during the menopausal transition in a population-based cohort of women. J Clin Endocrinol Metab. 1999;84:4025-30.
20. Seifer DB, Scott RT Jr, Bergh PA, Abrogast LK, Friedman CI, Mack CK, et al. Women with declining ovarian reserve may demonstrate a decrease in day 3 serum inhibin B before a rise in day 3 follicle-stimulating hormone. Fertil Steril. 1999;72:63-5.
21. Klein NA, Houmard BS, Hansen KR, Woodruff TK, Sluss PM, Bremner WJ, et al. Age-related analysis of inhibin A, inhibin B, and activin a relative to the intercycle monotropic follicle-stimulating hormone rise in normal ovulatory women. J Clin Endocrinol Metab. 2004;89:2977-81.
22. Hale GE, Zhao X, Hughes CL, Burger HG, Robertson DM, Fraser IS. Endocrine features of menstrual cycles in middle and late reproductive age and the menopausal transition classified according to the Staging of Reproductive Aging Workshop (STRAW) staging system. J Clin Endocrinol Metab. 2007;92:3060.
23. Knauff EA, Eijkemans MJ, Lambalk CB, ten Kate-Booij MJ, Hoek A, Beerendonk CC, et al. Anti-Müllerian hormone, inhibin B, and antral follicle count in young women with ovarian failure. J Clin Endocrinol Metab. 2009;94:786.
24. Burger HG, Hale GE, Dennerstein L, Robertson DM. Cycle and hormone changes during perimenopause: the key role of ovarian function. Menopause. 2008;15:603.
25. Welt CK, Smith ZA, Pauler DK, Hall JE. Differential regulation of inhibin A and inhibin B by luteinizing hormone, follicle-stimulating hormone, and stage of follicle development. J Clin Endocrinol Metab. 2001;86:2531.
26. Burger HG, Groome NP, Robertson DM. Both inhibin A and B respond to exogenous follicle-stimulating hormone in the follicular phase of the human menstrual cycle. J Clin Endocrinol Metab. 1998;83:4167.
27. Landgren BM, Collins A, Csemiczky G, Burger HG, Baksheev L, Robertson DM. Menopause transition: annual changes in serum hormonal patterns over the menstrual cycle in women during a nine-year period prior to menopause. J Clin Endocrinol Metab. 2004;89:2763.

28. Klein NA, Battaglia DE, Miller PB, Branigan EF, Giudice LC, Soules MR. Ovarian follicular development and the follicular fluid hormones and growth factors in normal women of advanced reproductive age. J Clin Endocrinol Metab. 1996;81:1946.
29. Welt CK, McNicholl DJ, Taylor AE, Hall JE. Female reproductive aging is marked by decreased secretion of dimeric inhibin. J Clin Endocrinol Metab. 1999;84:105.
30. de Koning CH, McDonnell J, Themmen AP, de Jong FH, Homburg R, Lambalk CB. The endocrine and follicular growth dynamics throughout the menstrual cycle in women with consistently or variably elevated early follicular phase FSH compared with controls. Hum Reprod. 2008;23:1416.
31. Miro F, Parker SW, Aspinall LJ, Coley J, Perry PW, Ellis JE. Sequential classification of endocrine stages during reproductive aging in women: the FREEDOM study. Menopause. 2005;12:281.
32. Mersereau JE, Evans ML, Moore DH, Liu JH, Thomas MA, Rebar RW, et al. Luteal phase estrogen is decreased in regularly menstruating older women compared with a reference population of younger women. Menopause. 2008;15:482.
33. Klein NA, Battaglia DE, Fujimoto VY, Davis GS, Bremmer WJ, Soules MR. Reproductive aging: accelerated ovarian follicular development associated with a monotropic follicle-stimulating hormone rise in normal older women. J Clin Endocrinol Metab. 1996;81:1038.
34. Soules MR, Sherman S, Parrott E, Rebar R, Santoro N, Utian W, et al. Executive summary: stages of reproductive aging workshop (STRAW). Fertil Steril. 2001;76:874.
35. den Tonkelaar I, te Velde ER, Looman CW. Menstrual cycle length preceding menopause in relation to age at menopause. Maturitas. 1998;29:115.
36. Weinstein M, Gorrindo T, Riley A, Mormino J, Niedfeldt J, Singer B, et al. Timing of menopause and patterns of menstrual bleeding. Am J Epidemiol. 2003;158:782.
37. Vollman RF. The menstrual cycle. In: Friedman E (Ed). Major Problems in Obstetrics and Gynecology. Philadelphia: W.B. Saunders Co; 1977.
38. Lisabeth L, Harlow S, Qaqish B. A new statistical approach demonstrated menstrual patterns during the menopausal transition did not vary by age at menopause. J Clin Epidemiol. 2004;57:484.
39. Broekmans FJ, Faddy MJ, Scheffer G, te Velde ER. Antral follicle counts are related to age at natural fertility loss and age at menopause. Menopause. 2004;11:607.
40. Kuliev A, Cieslak J, Verlinsky Y. Frequency and distribution of chromosome abnormalities in human oocytes. Cytogenet Genome Res. 2005;111:193.
41. Hunt PA, Hassold TJ, Human female meiosis: what makes a good egg go bad? Trends Genet. 2008;24:86.
42. Pellestor F, Anahory T, Hamamah S. Effect of maternal age on the frequency of cytogenetic abnormalities in human oocytes. Cytogenet Genome Res. 2005;111:206.
43. Jacobs SL, Metzger DA, Dodson WC, Haney AF. Effect of age on response to human menopausal gonadotropin stimulation. J Clin Endocrinol Metab. 1990;71:1525.
44. Nikolaou D, Templeton A. Early ovarian ageing: a hypothesis: detection and clinical relevance. Hum Reprod. 2003;18(6):1137-9.
45. Navot D, Bergh PA, Williams MA, Garrisi GJ, Guzman I, Sandler B, et al. Poor oocyte quality rather than implantation failure as a cause of age-related decline in female fertility. Lancet. 1991;337(8754):1375-7.

46. Liu L, Keefe DL. Ageing-associated aberration in meiosis of oocytes from senescence-accelerated mice. Hum Reprod. 2002;17(10):2678-85.
47. van Montfrans JM, van Hooff MH, Martens F, Lambalk CB. Basal FSH, estradiol and inhibin B concentrations in women with a previous Down's syndrome affected pregnancy. Hum Reprod. 2002;17(1):44-7.
48. Dorland M, van Kooij RJ, te Velde ER. General ageing and ovarian ageing. Maturitas. 1998;30(2):113-8.
49. Ossewaarde ME, Bots ML, Verbeek AL, Peeters PH, van der Graaf Y, Grobbee DE, et al. Age at menopause, cause-specific mortality and total life expectancy. Epidemiology. 2005;16(4):556-62.
50. Klein NA, Harper AJ, Houmard BS, Sluss PM, Soules MR. Is the short follicular phase in older women secondary to advanced or accelerated dominant follicle development? J Clin Endocrinol Metab. 2002;87:5746.
51. Hansen KR, Thyer AC, Sluss PM, Bremner WJ, Soules MR, Klein NA. Reproductive ageing and ovarian function: is the early follicular phase FSH rise necessary to maintain adequate secretory function in older ovulatory women? Hum Reprod. 2005;20:89.
52. Davison SL, Bell R, Donath S, Montalto JG, Davis SR. Androgen levels in adult females: changes with age, menopause, and oophorectomy. J Clin Endocrinol Metab. 2005;90(7):3847-53.
53. Dulitzki M, Soriano D, Schiff E, Chetrit A, Mashiach S, Seidman DS. Effect of very advanced maternal age on pregnancy outcome and rate of cesarean delivery. Obstet Gynecol. 1998;92(6):935-9.
54. Beemsterboer SN, Homburg R, Gorter NA, Schats R, Hompes PG, Lambalk CB. The paradox of declining fertility but increasing twinning rates with advancing maternal age. Hum Reprod. 2006;21:1531.
55. Hoekstra C, Zhao ZZ, Lambalk CB, Willemsen G, Martin NG, Boomsma DI, et al. Dizygotic twinning. Hum Reprod Update. 2008;14:37.
56. Wilcox AJ, Weiberg CR, O'Connor JF, Baird DD, Schlatterer JP, Canfield RE, et al. Incidence of early loss of pregnancy. N Engl J Med. 1988;319:189.
57. Zinaman MJ, Clegg ED, Brown CC, O'Connor J, Selevan SG. Estimates of human fertility and pregnancy loss. Fertil Steril. 1996;65:503.
58. Centers for Disease Control and Prevention, American Society for Reproductive Medicine, Society for Assisted Reproductive Technology. 2015 Assisted Reproductive Technology National Summary Report. Atlanta, (GA): US Dept of Health and Human Services; 2017.
59. Griffiths A, Dyer SM, Lord SJ, Pardy C, Fraser IS, Eckermann S. A cost-effectiveness analysis of in-vitro fertilization by maternal age and number of treatment attempts. Hum Reprod. 2010;25(4):924-31.
60. Reljič M, Lovrec VG. Predictive factors for live birth in autologous in vitro fertilization cycles in women aged 40 years and older. Zdr Varst. 2019;58(4):173-8.
61. Kalra SK, Ratcliffe SJ, Dokras A. Is the fertile window extended in women with polycystic ovary syndrome? Utilizing the Society for Assisted Reproductive Technology registry to assess the impact of reproductive aging on live-birth rate. Fertil Steril. 2013;100(1):208-13.
62. Haahr T, Dosouto C, Alviggi C, Esteves SC, Humaidan P. Management strategies for POSEIDON groups 3 and 4. Front Endocrinol. 2019;10:614.

Chapter 12

Current Concepts of Hormone Replacement Therapy

Ashwini Bhalerao Gandhi, Priya Vora, Rajeshwari Khyade

■ INTRODUCTION

Menopause is an important transition phase that brings in many changes that can affect the quality of a woman's life.[1] It is nature's protective phenomenon against reproductive morbidity and mortality in the aging population.[1] Due to the depletion of estrogen and progesterone from the aging, ovaries hormone therapy is administered in the form of synthetic estrogen and progesterone to replace a woman's depleting hormone levels, thus alleviating menopausal symptoms and preventing long-term adverse effects on bone, cardiovascular system, and urogenital system.

Hormone replacement therapy (HRT) underwent dramatic swings during the last 50 years. It was extremely popular before the Women's Health Initiative (WHI) study. The enthusiasm for HRT was smashed in 2002 after the WHI trial results, which stated that postmenopausal women taking combined hormone therapy had an increased risk for breast cancer, heart disease, stroke, and pulmonary emboli. After many years of debate between proponents and opponents of HRT and detailed analysis, HRT proved to be the most effective treatment for healthy women who experience troublesome menopausal symptoms when given for a limited period.

■ NEED FOR HORMONE REPLACEMENT THERAPY

The life expectancy of women in South Korea is predicted to rank first in the world by 2030, as it will reach to 90.82 years. In a recent study, it is estimated that worldwide 1 billion women by 2020[2] and 1.6 billion women by 2050 will be 50 years or older.[3] In India, the life expectancy of women is 72.3 years,[4] and the average age of attaining menopause is 47–49 years. Hence, maintaining a positive postreproductive phase, preventing noncommunicable diseases, reducing mortality, and improving quality of life after menopause are important.

In Indian women, the most common symptoms are vasomotor instability causing hot flashes, sweating, and palpitations. Urogenital symptoms such as urinary frequency, urgency, vaginal dryness, soreness, and dyspareunia are also frequent. Psychological symptoms such as mood changes, insomnia, depression, and anxiety make it difficult to cope in life. Long-term effects are osteoporosis, cardiovascular disease, and Alzheimer's disease. HRT also markedly reduces the other symptoms of menopause such as vasomotor, vaginal, and vulvar dryness, the risk of osteoporotic fractures, and overall improves the quality of life and well-being. Estrogen being lipid friendly increases high-density lipoprotein (HDL) and lowers low-density lipoprotein (LDL) cholesterol, prevents inflammatory changes, acts on smooth muscles, and causes vasodilation, thereby preventing atherosclerosis and cardiovascular accidents.[4] A study done by Zhang et al.[3] found that menopausal hormone therapy (MHT) was associated with decreased risk of cataract, glioma, and esophageal/gastric and colorectal cancers but increased risk of pulmonary embolism, cholelithiasis, asthma, meningioma and thyroid, breast, and ovarian cancer. He concluded that MHT has a complex balance of benefits and affects multiple health outcomes. In young healthy women (50–60 years old), the benefit outweighs the risks of using HRT.[5] Currently, the use of HRT is partly correlated with decreased incidence of lung cancer.[6] Danish Osteoporosis Prevention Study (DOPS)[7] and Kronos Early Estrogen Prevention Study (KEEPS)[8] concluded that MHT has a beneficial effect on coronary artery disease when initiated immediately after menopause.

■ WORKUP BEFORE HORMONE REPLACEMENT THERAPY

History-taking and a proper physical examination are essential. Complete blood count, blood sugars, liver function tests, lipid profile, and thyroid profile are important investigations needed to be performed. Pelvic ultrasonography, mammography, bone mineral density (BMD), Pap smear screening, etc., are helpful. Pre-MHT workup and annual follow-up are essential when prescribing MHT.

■ WHAT HAS CHANGED IN HORMONE REPLACEMENT THERAPY?

Estrogen in Menopausal Hormone Therapy

Conjugated equine estrogen (CEE) 0.3 mg/0.625 mg, estradiol valerate 1/2 mg, or 17β-estradiol 1 mg are present in the commonly used oral preparations. Nowadays, estrogen can be administered by other routes also; for example, transdermal patches, sprays, gels, topical emulsion preparations, and vaginal preparations are available. Risks of oral estrogens are from first-pass metabolism through the liver and include increased production of coagulation factors and various inflammatory markers, hypertriglyceridemia, and elevated risk of venous thromboembolism and gallstones. Transdermal and topical estrogens bypass first-pass metabolism and have the advantage of safety and accurate dosing. Transdermal therapy is preferred in case the patient is intolerant to oral therapy or in whom oral therapy is contraindicated. Transdermal estrogen sprays are also recently available. The maximum estradiol concentration is achieved 18–20 hours after application. A stable level reaches on the 7th–8th day of application.

Vaginal Estrogen

Low-dose vaginal estrogen therapy is approved by Food and Drug Administration (FDA) to treat moderate-to-severe vaginal dryness and dyspareunia caused by the genitourinary syndrome of menopause.

Vaginal creams, rings, tablets, or capsules are available in different countries. Its primary mechanism is to locally treat postmenopausal vulvovaginal changes. There are no systemic side effects with vaginal preparations. Also, addition of progesterone is not needed as there is no endometrial stimulation. Estriol and CEE creams are available. Ultra low-dose estriol 0.03 mg/day and standard dose 0.5 mg/day for 2 weeks followed by maintenance dose can be continued for a long time. But safety data beyond 1 year is unavailable.

Progesterone

The progesterone in the HRT also matters. Progestogen options include micronized progesterone and synthetic progestins, such as medroxyprogesterone acetate (MPA) or norethindrone. Micronized progesterone is bioidentical to the endogenous hormone and has efficient oral absorption. It can also be given vaginally. Compared to natural progesterone, synthetic progestins have 10–100-fold greater activity. Recently, combined preparations containing micronized progesterone or dydrogesterone are available. Progestogen therapy is primarily used to avoid an increased risk of endometrial cancer for a woman on systemic estrogen, as unopposed estrogen thickens the uterine lining and increases the risk of endometrial cancer. A woman who already has levonorgestrel-releasing intrauterine system (LNG-IUS) can be given oral or transdermal estrogens. LNG-IUS will give protection to the endometrium.

Selective estrogen receptor modulators (SERMS): SERMs are a category of drugs that act selectively as estrogen agonists or antagonists depending on the target tissue. *Tamoxifen, raloxifene, lasofoxifene, and bazedoxifene (BZA)* are SERMs used in different countries. They can be used in postmenopausal women of younger age, particularly in patients with a family history of invasive breast cancer as it reduces the incidence of this type of cancer.

Ospemifene: 60 mg daily significantly reduced the symptoms of dyspareunia and vaginal dryness compared with placebo in a randomized, 12-week multicenter, double-blind study. Percentages of superficial and parabasal cells improved along with the vaginal pH.[9]

Raloxifene is widely used for the prevention of osteoporosis.

Bazedoxifene is used in postmenopausal women for the prevention and treatment of osteoporosis. It is relatively safe and well tolerated. No breast or endometrial stimulation is found for the first 2 years. It increases endothelial nitric oxide synthase activity and does not antagonize the effects of 17β-estradiol on vasomotor symptoms (VMS). Combined estrogen with BZA is used in the treatment of moderate-to-severe VMS, prevention of postmenopausal osteoporosis, and treatment of estrogen deficiency symptoms in nonhysterectomized postmenopausal women. The combination allows the benefits of estrogen without estrogenic stimulation of the endometrium.

Lasofoxifene has a high affinity for both estrogen receptor α (ERα) and ERβ, the same as estradiol, and about 10 times higher than other SERMs. It is also highly selective, having >100-fold selectivity against other steroid receptors. In postmenopausal women with osteoporosis, lasofoxifene increased BMD at the lumbar spine and hip, reduced bone turnover, and reduced the risk of vertebral and nonvertebral fractures. It also decreased the risk of ER-positive breast cancer and improved the signs and symptoms of vulvovaginal atrophy. But it is associated with an increased incidence of hot flushes, venous thromboembolic events, vaginal bleeding, and muscle spasm. It is approved for postmenopausal women who are at an increased risk of fracture.[10]

Dehydroepiandrosterone

Dehydroepiandrosterone (DHEA) is FDA approved for genitourinary syndrome of menopause. According to the expert panel of the Polish Menopause and Andropause Society,[11] DHEA supplements are useful in postmenopausal women with hypoactive sexual disorders and in women with osteoporosis. In premenopausal women with sexual disorders and low libido, women with vulvovaginal atrophy, or genitourinary syndrome of menopause, DHEA can be used.[12]

MENOPAUSAL HORMONE THERAPY FORMULATIONS AVAILABLE IN INDIA (TABLE 1)

Estrogen
Oral—CEE 0.3 mg/0.625 mg, 17β-estradiol 1 mg/2 mg, estradiol valerate 1 mg/2 mg, and transdermal estrogen gel 0.125 mg/2.5 g of gel.

Progesterone
- Dydrogesterone 10 mg, micronized progesterone—100, 200, 300, 400 mg.
- Levonorgestrel intrauterine device—52 mg—releases 20 µg/day.

TABLE 1: Different formulations—estrogen and progestins.

Oral estrogen	Conjugated equine estrogen (CEE)	0.3 mg/0.625 mg
	17β-Estradiol	1 mg/2 mg body identical
Transdermal	17β-Estradiol estrogen gel	0.125 mg/2.5 g of gel Avoids first-pass metabolism
Oral progesterone	Norethindrone acetate	Indicated for abnormal uterine bleeding (AUB)
	Micronized progesterone	100, 200, 300, 400 mg body identical
	Medroxyprogesterone acetate	Strong action on the endometrium
	Dydrogesterone	10 mg
Intrauterine	Levonorgestrel	52 mg Releases 20 µg/day
Combination of estrogen and progesterone	17β-Estradiol and dydrogesterone	1 mg
Continuous sequential	17β-Estradiol and dydrogesterone	10 mg
Synthetic steroid	Tibolone	2.5 mg/day

Combination of Estrogen and Progesterone

- Combined sequential—17β-estradiol 1 and 10 mg of dydrogesterone.
- Continuous combined—17β-estradiol and dydrogesterone 5 mg daily.

Tibolone

Tibolone 2.5 mg/day orally is preferred to estrogen in women with poor sexual desire, mood swings, urogenital problems, fibroids, and high breast density.

ESTROGEN THERAPY FOR GENITOURINARY SYNDROME

- Estriol cream—0.5 mg/0.5 g of cream; oral estriol ½ mg.
- CEE—0.625 mg/1 g of cream.

CONTRAINDICATIONS FOR HORMONE REPLACEMENT THERAPY

Hormone therapy is contraindicated in patients with preexisting coronary heart disease, cerebrovascular disease, or thromboembolic tendencies. Before starting MHT, the symptoms can be reduced by lifestyle modifications such as weight loss, stress reduction, yoga, meditation, hypnosis, and cognitive behavioral therapy (CBT). Medications such as vitamin E, omega-3 fatty acids, isoflavones, and soya beans may be useful as MHT comes with its own risks and contraindications and should be given only when the benefits outweigh the risks. Therefore, MHT has to be started with a very low dose and for a minimum duration.[13] VMS normally appear within 1-2 years of the last menstruation and last for 4-5 years.

Low-dose MHT is more effective for treating VMS than the standard dose.[14] Symptomatic peri- and postmenopausal women and particularly those under 52 years, were more likely to have comorbid conditions such as depression, anxiety, osteoporosis, and insomnia.[15] Nonhormonal therapies, such as selective serotonin receptor inhibitors (SSRI) and selective norepinephrine receptor inhibitors (SNRI), showed a 40-65% reduction in these problems. Gabapentin 900 mg/day showed 50% reduction, and pregabalin 150 mg/day showed 65% improvement in VMS.[16,17]

■ GUIDELINES

According to National Institute for Health and Care Excellence (NICE) guidelines:[18]
- Offer women HRT for hot flushes and night sweats after discussing risks and benefits.
- Consider HRT to ease the mood and consider CBT to relieve low mood and anxiety.
- Estrogen alone has little or no increased risk of breast cancer. While estrogen and progesterone are associated with an increase in the risk of breast cancer, risk reduces after stopping HRT. HRT does not increase cardiovascular disease risk when started before 60 years of age. Refer the woman to a menopause specialist if there is no improvement.

International Menopause Society Guidelines[19]

According to International Menopause Society Guidelines:
- MHT is the most effective treatment for menopausal symptoms.
- MHT including tibolone and a combination of CEE and BZA is the most effective treatment for VMS associated with menopause.
- If MHT is not desired or contraindicated, SSRI and SNRI such as paroxetine, escitalopram, venlafaxine, desvenlafaxine, and gabapentin can be prescribed.
- MHT can be initiated in postmenopausal women at risk of fracture or osteoporosis before the age of 60 years or within 10 years of menopause.

2017 North American Menopausal Society Guidelines[20]

According to 2017 North American Menopausal Society guidelines:
- Treatment should be individualized to determine the most suitable type of hormone therapy. Dose, formulation, route of administration, and duration of use should be assessed and reassessed from time to time.

- A woman aged 60 years or older or who starts HRT after 10 years of onset of menopause has a greater risk of coronary heart disease, stroke, venous thromboembolism, and dementia. It makes the risks outweigh the benefits and hence is less favorable.
- For genitourinary symptoms, low-dose vaginal therapy or other therapies such as estrogen creams can be used.
- The latest evidence suggests that all women with VMS tend to have lower BMD and are at risk for osteoporosis.
- Women need to receive balanced and accurate information about the risk and benefits to make an informed choice before the start of MHT, as a range of treatment options are available for women who have symptoms.[21]
- MHT should not be used for the primary or secondary prevention of coronary heart disease.[22]
- There is no evidence for the efficacy of herbal supplements or acupuncture.

■ CONCLUSION

- Estrogen-containing products are widely used therapies for VMS and vaginal and vulvar atrophy.
- They are good for the prevention of osteoporosis, cardiovascular disease, and dementia, but they pose a serious risk of thromboembolism.
- Therefore, hormone therapy should be used at the lowest dose and for the shorter duration necessary to relieve the symptoms.
- Dose and duration should be tailor-made according to the patient's need and reviewed periodically.
- Low-dose regimens lower the risk of serious side effects.
- The patient should be counseled for lifestyle modifications and should try alternative therapies such as engaging in physical exercises, high-fiber diet intake, mindfulness techniques, yoga, and meditation.
- MHT should not be used for the primary or secondary prevention of coronary heart disease.

KEY MESSAGES

- Women should receive balanced and accurate information about the risks and benefits of hormone replacement therapy (HRT) to enable them to make an informed choice before the start of HRT.
- HRT should be used at the lowest dose and for the shortest duration necessary to relieve the symptoms. The risks are rare if given to women below 60 years of age or within 10 years of menopause.
- The dose and duration can be tailor-made according to the individual patient's need.
- Women should be counseled for suitable lifestyle modifications.
- HRT is contraindicated in women with preexisting hormone-dependent cancers/coronary heart disease, cerebrovascular disease, thromboembolic tendencies, or severe active liver disease.

Contd...

Contd…

- Oral, transdermal, and vaginal preparations are available. Oral preparations of estrogen can be combined with different types of progesterone such as medroxyprogesterone acetate (MPA), micronized progesterone, and dydrogesterone.
- Menopausal hormone therapy (MHT) covers therapies including estrogen, progestogens, combined therapies, androgens, and tibolone.
- Pre-MHT workup and annual follow-up are essential when prescribing MHT.
- Stopping MHT may be abrupt or the dose and duration may be tapered off gradually.

REFERENCES

1. Meeta M, Tandon V. Evidence-based clinical practice guidelines on menopause and postmenopausal osteoporosis (2019–2020): a step toward implementation of menopausal medicine. J Midlife Health. 2020;11(2):51-2.
2. Academic Committee of the Korean Society of Menopause, Lee SR, Cho MK, Cho YJ, Chun S, Hong SH, et al. The 2020 menopausal hormone therapy guidelines. J Menopausal Med. 2020;26(2):69-98.
3. Zhang GQ, Chen JL, Luo Y, Mathur MB, Anagnostis P, Nurmatov U, et al. Menopausal hormone therapy and women's health: an umbrella review. PLoS Med. 2021;18(8):e1003731.
4. Khadilkar SS. Post-reproductive health: window of opportunity for preventing comorbidities. J Obstet Gynaecol India. 2019;69(1):1-5.
5. Lobo RA. Hormone-replacement therapy: current thinking. Nat Rev Endocrinol. 2017;13:220-31.
6. Wen H, Lin X, Sun D. The association between different hormone replacement therapy use and the incidence of lung cancer: a systemic review and meta-analysis. J Thorac Dis. 2022;14(2):381-95.
7. Mosekilde L, Beck-Nielsen H, Sørensen OH, Nielsen SP, Charles P, Vestergaard P, et al. Hormonal replacement therapy reduces forearm fracture incidence in recent postmenopausal women—results of the Danish Osteoporosis Prevention Study. Maturitas. 2000;36(3):181-93.
8. Miller VM, Naftolin F, Asthana S, Black DM, Brinton EA, Budoff MJ, et al. The Kronos Early Estrogen Prevention Study (KEEPS): what have we learned? Menopause. 2019;26(9):1071-84.
9. Simon JA, Lin VH, Radovich C, Bachmann GA, Ospemifene Study Group. One-year long-term safety extension study of ospemifene for the treatment of vulvar and vaginal atrophy in postmenopausal women with a uterus. Menopause. 2013;20:418-27.
10. Lewiecki EM. Lasofoxifene for the prevention and treatment of postmenopausal osteoporosis. Ther Clin Risk Manag. 2009;5:817-27.
11. Rabijewski M, Papierska L, Binkowska M, Maksym R, Jankowska K, Skrzypulec-Plinta W, et al. Supplementation of dehydroepiandrosterone (DHEA) in pre- and postmenopausal women—position statement of an expert panel of Polish Menopause and Andropause Society. Ginekol Pol. 2020;91(9):554-62.

12. Labrie F, Archer DF, Koltun W, Vachon A, Young D, Frenette L, et al. Efficacy of intravaginal dehydroepiandrosterone (DHEA) on moderate-to-severe dyspareunia and vaginal dryness, symptoms of vulvovaginal atrophy, and of the genitourinary syndrome of menopause. Menopause. 2016;23(3):243-56.
13. Banks NK. Practice essentials. In: Richard Scott (Ed). Menopausal Hormone Replacement Therapy. Medscape; 2021.
14. Akhila V, Pratapkumar. A comparison of transdermal and oral HRT for menopausal symptom control. Int J Fertil Womens Med. 2006;51:64-9.
15. Sharman Moser S, Chodick G, Bar-On S, Shalev V. Healthcare utilization and prevalence of symptoms in women with menopause: a real-world analysis. Int J Womens Health. 2020;12:445-54.
16. Espeland MA, Rapp SR, Shumaker SA, Brunner R, Manson JE, Sherwin BB, et al. Conjugated equine estrogen and global cognitive function in postmenopausal women: Women's Health Initiative Memory Study. JAMA. 2004;291(24):2959-68.
17. Zandi PP, Carlson MC, Plassman BL, Welsh-Bohmer KA, Mayer LS, Steffens DC, et al. Hormone replacement therapy and incidence of Alzheimer disease in older women: the Cache County Study. JAMA. 2002;288(17):2123-9.
18. National Collaborating Centre for Women's and Children's Health (UK). Menopause. London: National Institute for Health and Care Excellence; 2015.
19. de Villiers TJ, Hall JE, Pinkerton JV, Cerdas Pérez S, Rees M, Yang C, et al. Revised Global Consensus Statement on Menopausal Hormone Therapy. Climacteric. 2016;19(4):313-5.
20. The NAMS 2017 Hormone therapy Position Statement Advisory Panel. The 2017 Hormone Therapy Position Statement of the North American Menopause Society. Menopause. 2017;24(7):728-53.
21. Magrait K, Stuckey B. Making choices at menopause. Aust J Gen Pract. 2019;48(7):457-2.
22. Boardman HM, Hartley L, Eisinga A, Main C, Roqué i Figuls M, Bonfill Cosp X, et al. Hormone therapy for preventing cardiovascular disease in post-menopausal women. Cochrane Database Syst Rev. 2015;(3):CD002229.

Index

Page numbers followed by *b* refer to box, *f* refer to figure, *fc* refer to flowchart, and *t* refer to table.

A

Abdominal girth 92
   monitoring of 91
Adenomyosis 66
Adenosine triphosphate 9
   production of 102
Adrenal hyperandrogenemia 4
Albumin 89
Alzheimer's disease 128
Amenorrhea 3, 97
   secondary 97
Androgens 35, 103
   role of 32
Androstenedione 9, 118
Anklesaria's Indian Menopause Society consensus group staging, modified 81*t*
Anovulation, chronic 47
Anti-centromere antibody 99
Anti-Müllerian hormone 2, 3, 22, 33, 38, 50, 51, 53, 55, 67, 80, 97, 101
   levels 68
   role of 33, 33*f*
   serum 22, 67
Antral follicle 9, 15, 29
   count 2, 3, 22, 23, 38, 51, 53, 55, 78, 86, 119, 120*f*
Anxiety 82
Appendicitis 91
Aromatase
   deficiency 98
   inhibitors 53, 89
Aspirin 88
Assisted reproductive technology 53, 66, 68, 119
Asthma 128
Ataxia 98
   telangiectasia 118
Atresia 2, 106
Autoimmune polyglandular syndrome 98

B

Basal endocrine assays 119
Basal serum follicle-stimulating hormone 21
Bazedoxifene 129, 130
Biochemical androgen excess 28
Biophysical tests 119
Biopsy, ovarian 24
Blastocyst transfer, proportion of 119
Blepharophimosis 98
Blood, ovarian 3
Bloom syndrome 98
Body
   mass index 4, 47, 82, 86
   weight, monitoring of 91
Bone morphogenetic protein 101
Breast 128
   cancer 127
Breath, shortness of 92

C

Calcium 104
   gluconate 89
Cancer
   ovarian 128
   types of 129
Cardiovascular disease 82, 128
   development of 82
Cholelithiasis 128
Chromium 62
   poly-nicotinate 62
Clomiphene citrate 39, 41, 41*f*
   challenge test 3, 23
Coenzyme Q10 63, 102
Cognitive behavioral therapy 131
Controlled ovarian hyperstimulation 38
   disadvantages of 44
Controlled ovarian stimulation 67, 73, 87, 116
Corpus luteum
   formation 114
   maintenance of 1
Cortex specific stroma, loss of 68
C-reactive protein 90
Cyclic adenosine monophosphate 4, 9
Cyclic follicle maturation 114
Cyclic guanosine monophosphate 4
Cysts 74
   bilateral 74
   rupture 91
Cytomegalovirus 98

Index

D

Dehydroepiandrosterone 31, 52, 102, 130
    sulfate 118
Deliveries, premature 44
Deoxyribonucleic acid 102
Diabetes mellitus 60
Dominant follicle 42
    selection of 7*f*
Dopamine agonists 89
Double ovarian stimulation 52, 72
Down syndrome 118
Dydrogesterone 130
    molecule 73
Dynorphin 13, 14
    role of 13
Dyspareunia 127

E

Electrolyte imbalance management 89
Embryos 20, 118
    fertilized 66
    freezing of 88
Endocrine gland, temporary 13
Endometrioma 67, 70
Endometriosis 40, 66, 67, 69, 70, 72
    advanced 66, 69, 70, 73
    fertility index 66
    grades of 71
    mild-to-minimal 73
    severe 68, 73
Enzyme acetyl-CoA carboxylase 60
Equine estrogen, conjugated 128
Estradiol 3, 11, 79
    serum 21
Estrogen 5, 128, 130, 131
    low levels of 5
    microenvironment 10
    oral 131
    receptor alpha 130
    replacement therapy 117
    synthesis 103
    therapy 131
Euglycemia 59
European Society of Human Reproduction and Embryology Bologna Consensus 50
Exogenous follicle-stimulating hormone ovarian reserve test 3, 23

F

Fanconi anemia 98
Fertility 78
    natural 122
    precedes, loss of 115
    preservation 102
    rates 115
    treatment for 102, 120
Fluid management 92
Folic acid 63
Follicle 116
    depletion, rate of 115
    development of 7, 107
    preovulatory 12*fc*, 15
    recruitment 8
    reserve 115
    stimulating hormone 1, 3, 6, 9, 11, 30, 33, 38, 41*f*, 42, 42*f*, 44, 46, 51, 61, 78-80, 87, 103, 117
        functions of 4
        receptor 54, 103
        recombinant 54, 121
Follicular
    fluid 62
    growth, stages of 29*f*
    maturation, induction of 45
    phase 11*f*
    recruitment 7
Folliculogenesis 29, 79
Frozen embryo 71

G

Galactosemia 98
Genitourinary syndrome, estrogen therapy for 131
Germ cells 114
    mitotic multiplication of 114
    number of 114
    store of 114
Glands, pituitary 1
Gonadotropin 29*f*, 41, 42, 47
    disadvantages of 40
    preparations 41
    protocol 41
    releasing hormone 1, 3, 12, 52, 69, 86, 116
        agonist 3, 23, 46, 54, 55, 70
        analogs 46*f*
        antagonist 46, 47, 71, 87
    role of 40
    side effects of 44
    therapy 44, 45, 47
    use of 40
Graafian 29
Granulosa cells 9, 10, 30, 31, 33, 114
    aromatase activity 32
    mass of 12

H

Heart disease 127
   coronary 133
Hemoglobin, glycated 60
Hemorrhage, postpartum 103
High-dose gonadotropin stimulation 86
Hormone
   replacement therapy 104, 127, 128, 131, 133
      current concepts of 127
      need for 127
   therapy 131
      combined 127
Hot flashes, lower rates of 82
Human chorionic gonadotropin 41-44, 86, 99, 121
   avoidance of 88
Human granulosa cells 89
Human menopausal gonadotropin 41, 41f, 71, 121
Hutchison-Gilford progeria 118
Hyaluronic acid 105
Hydroxyethyl starch 89
Hydroxylase 99
Hyperandrogenemia 28
Hyperandrogenism 28
Hyperinsulinemia 59
Hyperkalemia 90
Hyperprolactinemia 4, 38
Hyponatremia 90
Hypothalamic-pituitary
   abnormalities 59
   gonadal axis 3
   ovarian axis 1

I

In vitro
   activation 104
   fertilization 20, 50, 67, 70, 89, 118
   maturation 89
Infection, pelvic 91
Infertility
   causes of 38
   duration of 66
   treatment of 40
Inhibin-activin-follistatin system 6
Insomnia rates 82
Insulin 35
   role of 32
International Menopause Society Guidelines 132
Intracytoplasmic sperm injection 50, 70
Intrafollicular melatonin concentrations 62
Intrauterine 131
   growth restriction 103
   insemination 40, 41
      ovarian stimulation for 46
Intrinsic dysfunction 32
Intrinsic mesenchymal-epithelial cell interactions 29

K

Kisspeptin 13
   role of 13
   trigger 90
Kronos Early Estrogen Prevention Study 128

L

Lasofoxifene 129, 130
Last menstrual period 35
Letrozole 39, 40, 53
Levonorgestrel intrauterine device 129, 130
Lipoprotein
   high-density 128
   low-density 128
Live birth rate 119
   cumulative 51
Liver function tests 90
L-methyl folate 63
Low molecular weight heparin 91
Low-dose vaginal estrogen therapy 129
Luteal estradiol priming 52
Luteal follicular transition 13, 16
Luteal gonadotropin stimulation 53
Luteal phase 13
   deficiency 3
   ovarian stimulation 72
   stimulation protocols 71
   support 73
Luteinizing hormone 1, 3, 6, 9, 11f, 12, 28, 46, 51, 72, 116, 121
   effect of 11f
   functions of 4
   recombinant 54
   role of 13
   surge, premature 45

M

Malaria 98
Medroxyprogesterone acetate 129
Melatonin 62

Index

Meningioma 128
Menopausal hormone therapy 128
    formulations 130
Menopausal symptoms 78, 79
Menopausal transition
    early 79
    late 79
Menopause 2, 78, 102, 115, 115*f*, 127
    age of 115
    genitourinary syndrome of 129
    transition
        menstrual irregularity of 79
        period 78
Menstrual abnormalities 98
Menstrual bleeding 88
Menstrual cycle 2, 6*f*, 79
    natural 7
    phases of 4
    physiology of 3
Menstrual irregularity 79
Messenger ribonucleic acid 101
Metabolic syndrome 60
Metformin 60, 61
    therapy 87
Micro-ribonucleic acid 103, 107
Miscarriage 44
    spontaneous 118
Mood changes 82
Mumps oophoritis 98
Myoinositol 61

N

N-acetylcysteine 62
Neurokinin B 13, 14
    role of 13
Neuropeptides 13
Non-assisted reproductive technology
        cycles 38
Noncommunicable diseases 127
Normal follicles, atresia of 106

O

Oligoanovulation 28
Oocyte 1, 30, 104, 116
    depletion of 2
    donation 73, 103
        conceptions 103
    maturation 62
    quality 51, 70, 116, 122
        measure of 24
    secreted factors 29
    store of 114
Oogonia 2

Oophoritis, autoimmune 117
Organ perfusion 92
Ospemifene 129
Osteoporosis 128, 130
    postmenopausal 130
Ovarian aging
    consequences of 118
    early 117
Ovarian cycle 6*f*
    pituitary 5
Ovarian dysfunction 59
Ovarian follicle 14, 106
    cohort 79
    granulosa cells of 21
Ovarian fossa 105
Ovarian hormonal levels 6
Ovarian hyperstimulation syndrome 39,
        43, 44, 86, 93
    complications of 89
    low risk of 87
    management of 86
    mild-moderate 91
    moderate-to-severe 86
    prevention of 86, 88
    risk factors for 86
    severity of 93
    treatment of 89
Ovarian insufficiency
    premature 97, 100*t*, 102, 103, 106,
        117, 117*t*
    primary 99
Ovarian paracrine activity 118
Ovarian reserve 1, 47, 120
    diminished 97
    test 3*fc*, 20, 21*b*, 24, 25, 50
Ovarian response 50, 68
Ovarian stimulation 38, 46, 66, 69, 70, 97
    response 86
Ovarian suppression, role of 68
Ovarian tissue 73, 105
    cryopreservation 102
Ovarian torsion 91
Ovarian volume 3, 24
    low 121*f*
Ovary 114
    normal 29
Ovulation 12
    induction 38, 45
        agents 39
        protocols 41
    physiology of 1
Ovulatory dysfunction 28
Ovulogens, oral 39
Oxidative stress 88

Index

P

Pain, abdominal 92
Paracentesis 92
Pelvic abscess 91
Perimenopausal period 81
Phosphoinositide 3-kinase 8*fc*
Pituitary luteinizing hormone 87
Platelet-rich plasma
    intraovarian infusion 106
    mechanisms of 106
    therapy
        countermeasures of 107
        risk of 107
Polycystic ovarian
    disease 59
    morphology 28, 31*f*, 34*b*
    syndrome 4, 24, 28, 47, 53, 59, 86
Polycystic ovary 30
    pathophysiology of 33*f*
Poor oocyte quality 24
POSEIDON classification 51, 51*b*, 55
Postmenopause
    early 79
    late 81
Preantral follicles 29
Prediabetes 60
Pregnancy 93
    confirmation of 88
    multiple 86
    rates 73
        clinical 97
        cumulative 119
    spontaneous 102
Preimplantation genetic
    screening 55
    testing 73
Premature ovarian insufficiency 97, 100*t*, 102, 103, 106, 117, 117*t*
    biomaterial strategies for 106
    causes of 98
    diagnosis of 102
    evaluation of 99
    iatrogenic risk for 97
    innovative therapeutic options for 104
    management of 104, 105*f*
    treatment 104
        future direction of 107
Primordial follicles 29, 115, 115*f*
    activation of 8
Progesterone 11*f*, 12, 45, 72, 129-131
    natural 129
    oral 131
Progestins, oral 73
Protein kinase B 8
Psychological distress, prevalence of 82

R

Raloxifene 129, 130
Receptor tyrosine kinase 8
Red blood cell 105
Reproductive stage, late 78
Ribonucleic acid 101

S

Selective estrogen receptor modulator 39, 129
Selective serotonin receptor inhibitors 132
Sex
    hormone-binding globulin 61
    steroids, secretion of 1
Sleep 82
Soreness 127
Spindle-shaped pregranulosa cells 114
Squamous granulosa cells 29
Stem cell
    adipose-derived 106
    adult 105
    embryonic 105
    pluripotent 105
    therapy 105
    transplantation 106
Steroid
    hormone concentrations 14
    metabolism 31*f*
    ovarian 14
Steroidogenesis 9
    ovarian 28
Stimulation strategies 54
Straw staging system 78
Stroke 127
Supplementation therapy 53
Surgery, role of 69

T

Tamoxifen 39-41, 129
Telangiectasia 98
Testosterone 61, 118
    gel 103
Thoracentesis 92
Threonine protein kinase 8, 8*fc*
Thromboprophylaxis 92

Index

Thyroid 128
    autoimmunity 117
    peroxidase antibody 99
    stimulating hormone 38, 61
Tibolone 131
Toxic chemicals 106
Transvaginal ultrasonography 22
Tuberculosis 98
Turner syndrome 98
Two-gonadotropin theory 9, 9*f*, 103

U

Ultralong gonadotropin-releasing hormone agonist protocol 71
Ultrasonography 41
Urinary tract infection 98
Uterine malformation 66

V

Vaginal dryness 82, 127
    moderate-to-severe 129
Vaginal estrogen 129
Varicella 98
Vascular endothelial dysfunction 92
Vascular endothelial growth factor 67, 87
    antagonists 90
Vasomotor symptoms 81, 130
    moderate-to-severe 130
Vitamin
    B_9 63
    D 61
        supplements 104

W

Werner syndrome 118